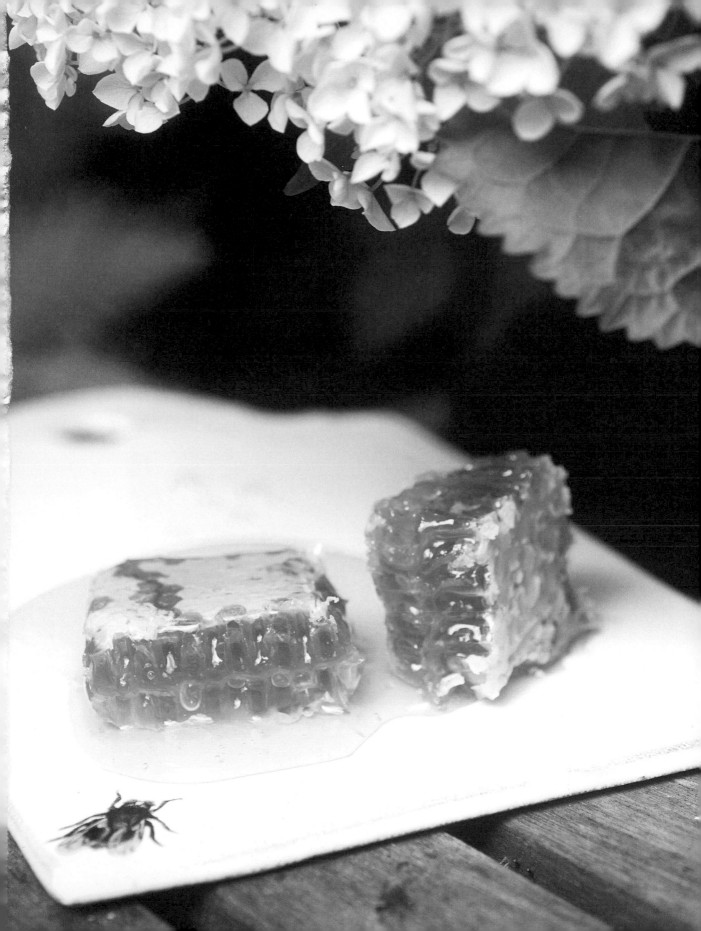

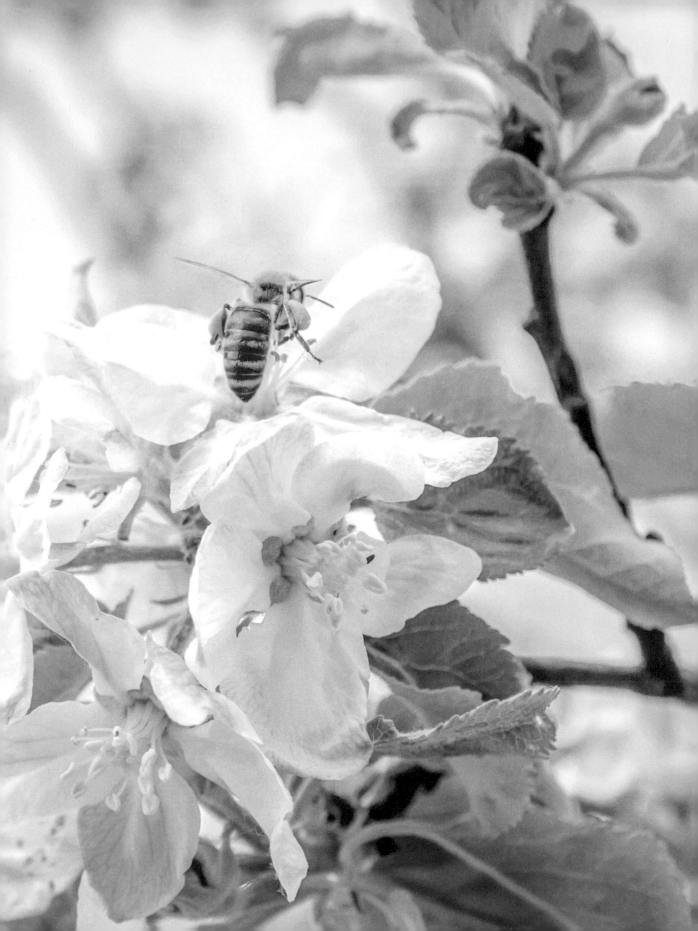

FERTILE

Nourish and Balance
Your Body Ready
for Baby Making

EMMA CANNON

WITH VICTORIA WELLS

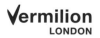
Vermilion
LONDON

10 9 8 7 6 5 4 3 2 1

Vermilion, an imprint of Ebury Publishing,
20 Vauxhall Bridge Road,
London SW1V 2SA

Vermilion is part of the Penguin Random House group
of companies whose addresses can be found at
global.penguinrandomhouse.com

 Penguin
Random House
UK

First published in the United Kingdom by
Vermilion in 2017

www.penguin.co.uk

A CIP catalogue record for this book is available from
the British Library

ISBN 9781785040894

Printed and bound in China by
C&C Offset Printing Co., Ltd

Penguin Random House is committed to a sustainable
future for our business, our readers and our planet.
This book is made from Forest Stewardship Council®
certified paper.

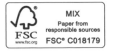

MIX
Paper from
responsible sources
FSC® C018179

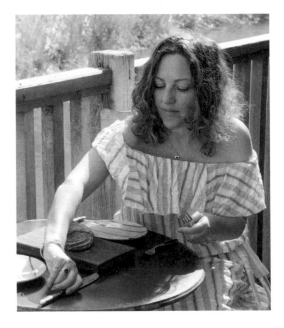

Contents

Introduction

> **Fertile** (*definition*): [1] The willingness and ability to receive:
> love, nutrition, abundance, nourishment, creativity, kindness,
> wonder, a new way of being. [2] The ability to conceive; to create
> a new life. [3] Rich in resources, fruitful and prolific.

This is a book to help you to live a more fertile life. A book to help you engage in your health and fertility so that when you are ready to have a baby you will be as fertile as possible. Being healthy and being fertile go hand in hand.

This book is as much for your heart as it is for your body. It is a book about passion – passion for life and passion for food. I will show you how to live a more fertile, balanced and abundant life, without losing the joy. I will teach you how to really nourish yourself and your loved ones, both by helping you to understand what your body needs and by offering up a whole selection of tasty, nutritious recipes in the second half of this book. As I always say, if you want to nourish another, first you must learn to nourish yourself.

This book is about making delicious food and still leaving time for baby making. After all, you can have the best diet in the world but if you don't find time for making love, babies tend to take a lot longer to put in an appearance. Pleasure, emotion and creation are intrinsically linked; keep that in mind when you start thinking about making a baby.

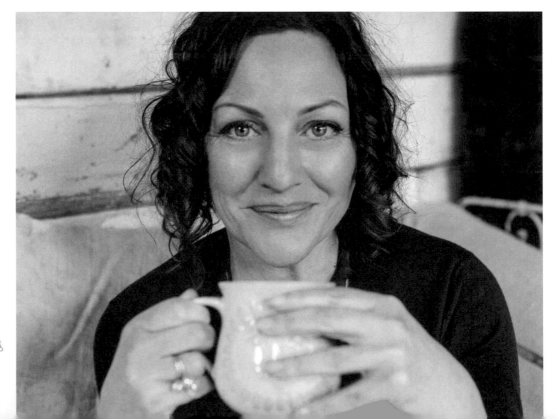

INTRODUCTION

I will show you how to understand your body, what to eat to make your body function better and maintain a healthy weight, how to improve digestion and gut microbes, how to use food to manage minor (and not so minor) period problems, how to give yourself a monthly tonic, how to live to be more fertile, and how to have balanced hormones, manage your mood swings and improve your libido.

While I have studied many different systems of medicine, my original training was in tongue and pulse and differential diagnosis. These techniques are all part of Chinese medicine diagnosis and I use them on every patient. Differential diagnosis is a process of history taking that allows me to gain a unique insight into the person's individual energetic picture and enables me to treat every patient appropriately and differently. Same disease; different patient! In other words, three people may have endometriosis but it will manifest differently in each person, meaning that each patient will need a different approach. It is fascinating to me that Western medicine is coming round to this approach, which they refer to as 'individualised treatments', but it has always been part of ancient systems of medicine such as Chinese medicine and Ayurvedic medicine.

I cannot imagine treating any other way and this is why this book is not like any other book you may read on diet, where everyone is recommended to eat the same foods. In my mind, this could never work; we are not all the same, we all respond to things in a different way, and have different constitutions and our own internal climate (which I tell you about in detail in Fertile Food, *see pages 27–42*). All of this means that we respond to food, medicine, alcohol, stimulants, environment, emotions, illness and stress in an entirely unique way. So rule one is never compare yourself to anyone else – it is pointless!

My aim with this book is to enable you to come as close to the experience of a visit to my clinic as possible, and that means adapting my advice to fit your individual situation. This needs to work with your life and it needs to work for you. Of course, I am not actually there with you so I can't make it bespoke for you. So you will need to develop some intuition. I don't want you to follow what I suggest slavishly and create a joyless life for yourself. A fertile approach to living has joy at the heart of it. So if you are taking what I say in a rigid and controlled way, put the book down, go for a walk and listen to the voice inside you. This will take practice because I am not talking about the Mind here, I am talking Heart. When I listen to my patients in clinic, I hear what they are saying, but I also listen to what they are not telling me – I listen with my heart. Practise what I call 'the middle way'; listen to my advice, but make it work for you.

I'd like to offer a little guidance around modern self-help approaches, diet and psychotherapy. I am a big fan of positive mental attitude and personal responsibility, often through modern self-help approaches, diet and psychotherapy. I believe it is important for us to develop awareness and to address past issues that may prevent us from being happy and healthy in the present. Emotions do impact on our physical health and they are not separate, the emotional backdrop to a person's life must always be considered and not to do so is neglectful.

However, I have seen an increased number of people taking it all a little bit too far; taking responsibility and blaming themselves when things go wrong. 'I feel like I am not getting pregnant because when I was trying to be positive some doubts crept in,' or 'I think the coffee I drank caused the miscarriage,' or 'I had a termination years ago and this is my punishment.' When things go wrong in life we have not always caused them by our thoughts and our actions, nor is the universe punishing us for something we have or have not done. Punishing yourself for not eating an entirely perfect diet or not having entirely pure and positive thoughts one hundred per cent of the time is a tension in and of itself. Take the middle road, find your own balance, do not punish yourself or blame yourself for things that may be out of your control. Be content with being 'good enough'.

Throughout this book I have included some very basic principles of Chinese medicine and some terminology that will help you. I have tried to strike a balance between giving you enough information and not baffling you! Actually, although I am simplifying it here for the sake of ease, Chinese medicine is an extremely complex system of healing with thousands of years of history. I hope I do not do it a disservice by diluting it down to the very simple version in this book. This is never my intention, but in order to keep this elegant medicine current I feel that it must also change and progress much like Western medicine does.

This system of medicine is able to address so many modern-day ills that were not even in existence when it was first developed. I am always in awe of the insights that I get from some of the very basic principles I was taught more than 20 years ago and I remain engaged and inspired by this beautiful medicine. Yet it is not perfect – no system is – and I find it works best when combined with Western medicine and a whole body approach, drawing on other ideas I have gleaned from yoga, psychotherapy, herbalism, modern nutritional and lifestyle research and through years of clinical observation of patients.

My aim is always to help you cultivate health and fertility, without becoming rigid or controlling. I want you to be consciously engaged in your health and the fertile choices you make every day. In many ways, baby making is a lot like cooking. First, we must have all the right ingredients and a vision of what we are trying to create. Next, we have to put the ingredients together, with good timing, and then we wait for the transformation to occur. When we bake a cake, at some point we must leave it alone and not keep looking and poking and prodding. So we can prepare and do our very best, and then the moment must come when we feel ready to have faith in the process, sit back and let the magic happen.

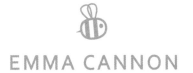

EMMA CANNON

A FERTILE LIFE

When you tend to a garden you don't seek to control it; take the same approach with your body and menstrual cycle. Tend to your body tenderly, without trying to control it.

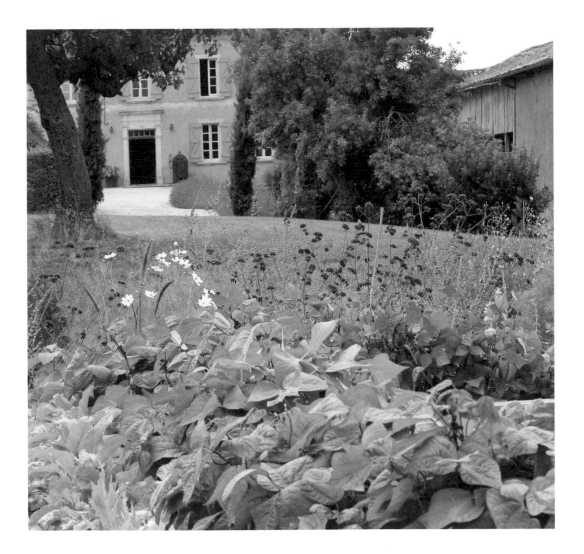

The five ingredients of a fertile life

Flexibility   Creativity   Nourishment   Transformation   Belief

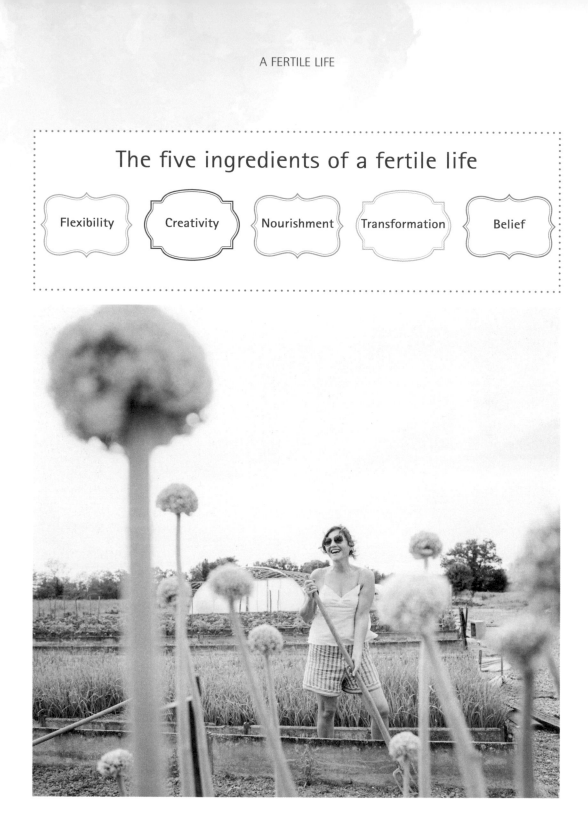

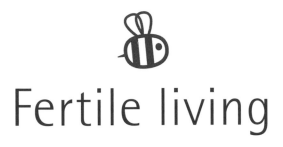

Fertile living

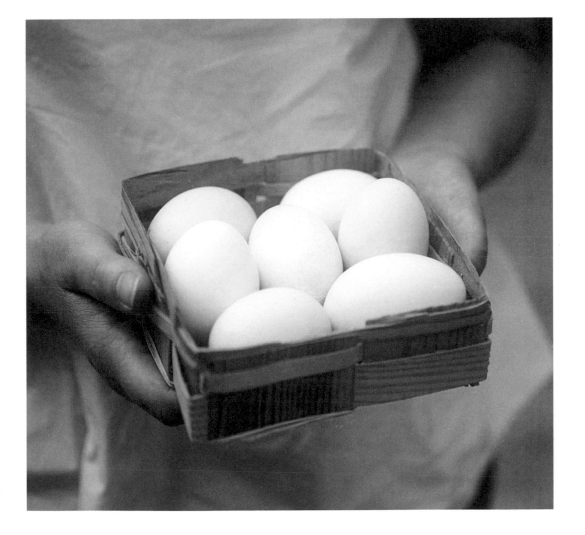

Throughout our day, however busy we are, there are tiny adjustments that can be made to live a more fertile life. These can be as simple as getting up 20 minutes earlier to stretch or meditate or to spend 20 minutes on a heartfelt project that always gets put to the bottom of the 'to do' list. Or deciding to engage fully in making a delicious breakfast to start the day, instead of reaching for empty calories; or walking to work and taking in our surroundings; or being engaged and focused in what we are doing instead of what we could be doing or what we will be doing later. 'Be here now,' I often remind my patients – and myself! Be present; enjoy the moment for what it is. This is where happiness lies, not in something not yet achieved. We are all busy but small adjustments can bring great changes.

Living a fertile life means being honest about how you really want to spend your precious time. For you, this might be leaving work on time and not feeling guilty, or saying 'no' when you mean 'no', instead of saying 'yes' and not meaning it. It is about feeling joyful about food and making choices that will preserve and optimise your fertility, your health and your wellbeing for many years to come.

In the twenty-first century we are living longer and have higher expectations than ever before of what our bodies ought to be able to achieve. I have discovered that it doesn't matter what reason a new patient or couple has for coming to see me, my role is to help them be more balanced, whether it is in the body, the mind or in their lives (usually it is in a little of all three). It is encouraging to see so many people now actively involved in their own health and fertility. The conversation is really beginning to grow around this topic and people appear to be more able to talk openly about fertility. Concerns about not leaving it too late to conceive and also how diet or lifestyle might have an impact on fertility are all current topics of discussion. There is a real sea change in people's awareness and an acceptance that how we live our lives does impact on our health and fertility.

Jing (essence)

Jing is the term used in Chinese medicine to describe our Essence, or constitutional health. Jing is a fundamental aspect of fertility and long life and it determines our individual reproductive capabilities. In many ways this book is based on ways to nourish and protect Jing so that you are able to remain in optimal fertility for as long as your individual constitution determines.

The health of the parents at the time of conception determines the health of the child. Some people are born with plentiful Jing inherited from their parents and others inherit less. Parents with good Jing tend to pass this on to their children, unless there is trauma in pregnancy or in birth. Good living can go some way to preserving and optimising Jing. So even those who are born with less Jing may be able to improve it by good lifestyle choices, whereas those with poor Jing and who make poor lifestyle choices may weaken their fertility for ever. Poor living, overworking, not recovering from illness and trauma and accidents can all deplete our Jing.

Our Jing is unique to us, so it is completely pointless comparing ourselves to others. So often patients will say to me, 'but so and so ran marathons right up until she had her baby and she was fine,' or 'Victoria Beckham was stick thin when she conceived', or 'my husband won't give up drinking because his friend Harry drank like a fish and Mary still conceived even though she smoked 20 cigarettes a day'. This sort of talk is completely futile as it is all a matter of individual reproductive capabilities – not to mention the fact that Harry and Mary's child may not have been particularly healthy!

Our mothers

While we are on the subject of Jing, our constitutional inheritance, it is a good time to think about your mum. Our biological mothers hold a great deal of important information for us regarding our own health. If you are lucky enough to have your mum around, make sure you have a chat with her. Find out if she had any gynaecological problems, what age she was when she had the menopause, whether she smoked when pregnant with you or if she had any major health issues around your birth or conception. It is all useful information when assessing your own potential powers of fertility.

My family

In my house food is the first medicine. I use food to keep my family healthy and to manage minor health problems. When my children seem under the weather or are getting a cold and producing lots of phlegm I immediately make a chicken broth and send them to bed early. Then I simplify their diet by removing all phlegm-forming foods and including foods that eliminate phlegm. Neither of my children has ever needed antibiotics or any medication for that matter. Not that I wouldn't give it to them; I am very pragmatic about these things. But I have always managed to keep them well with food, rest and occasionally a little acupuncture. In fact when Lily, my eldest, went to university the nurse could not believe that she had never had need for medication! The most emotional part of dropping her off was visiting the university canteen where I shed a tear knowing that she would need to fend for herself nutritionally now and all I could do was hope that I had steered her in the right direction.

Why this book is different

When I read other books I am amazed at how they are written as if we are all the same and we all need to eat the same foods in order to be healthy. Of course, there are some basic truths about what constitutes a healthy diet: more vegetables, less sugar, fewer refined foods, less meat, some fish and so on. But none of the health food books on the market considers the individual needs of the person. I believe that 'one man's meat is another man's poison'. In other words, we all benefit from slightly different approaches. That doesn't mean that everyone should sit down with an entirely different meal, but small adjustments can be made to make a dish more or less beneficial to the individual. This book is divided into two parts. The first half of the book covers everything you need to know to engage with your unique body and maximise your fertility. The second half contains delicious, fertility-boosting recipes. Throughout the book you will learn how you can adjust the food you prepare to make it as nutritious and fertility enhancing as possible for you and for your partner.

How to use this book

There are many different ways to use this book depending on your needs. I have made it as close to the experience of coming to my clinic as possible; everyone is different and needs a personal approach. In this case YOU decide, under my guidance, what you need and what feels right. I really want you to develop self-awareness and go with your gut instinct. Be your own guru!

All the recipes included in the book are good for everybody, but we have included notes so that you can tweak the recipe with an added ingredient to be even more beneficial to your individual needs. That way both you and your partner can eat and enjoy food together which, after all, is much more important than agonising over what you can and cannot eat. The bottom line is that everything in this book is good, wholesome, fertile food. Make sure your attitude towards it is the same; there is little more damaging to the body and mind than an unhealthy relationship with the very things that nourish us.

You can take a simple approach and just dip in and out of the recipes; cook whatever makes your heart sing and tune in to what your body is telling you and how you respond to certain foods. Listen to your body and, before you eat, think about what you are about to consume and whether or not it feels right. Alternatively, follow one of the programmes below, or be guided by the chapter that relates to your particular situation.

Assessing your tendencies

Use the self-assessment section (*see pages 28–37*) to decide what your tendencies are and how to balance your internal climate. I think this is useful for everyone. Even if you don't fully identify with one type, the exercise will make you more body aware. For example, you may identify in some respects with Blood Deficiency, in which case you need to include lots of recipes and foods that nourish Blood (*see page 33*). I would like you to use this knowledge as gentle background information. Most people will identify with many of the tendencies and climates – that's perfect. But some of you will feel you very much identify with one in particular. Also fine, but perhaps you will benefit from trying to balance out your tendencies. Whether or not you strongly resonate with a particular tendency is not important. What matters is that by looking at the tendencies you will start to engage with your body in a more fertile way. Do not be too rigid with it.

The Fertile Cleanse

The Fertile Cleanse (*see pages 59–68*) is good to do in the Spring, or as a preparation to getting started if you are hoping to get pregnant soon, or before IVF. It gives you an opportunity to make a change and improve your eating habits. I want to avoid words like 'good' and 'bad', 'clean' and 'dirty' in connection with food. I think these words are too emotive to use and I don't want to encourage anyone to be virtuous about food. For me there is as much dysfunction in virtue as there is in sloth! We are looking for a balanced approach.

The Menstrual Tonic

The Menstrual Tonic (*see pages 52–54*) is a lovely practice for any woman who wishes to engage with her monthly cycle and use food to enhance the natural rhythm of the body. It is suitable for women in their teens and twenties as well as older women, and you do not need to be trying for a baby to experience the benefits; it can just be a lovely self-care ritual. I suggest doing the tonic after the Fertile Cleanse. It is something I have used for many years in clinic and it is very powerful in helping women not only to engage with their bodies but to regulate their hormones throughout the month. You can do it every month if you really love it and are actively trying for a baby, or four times a year as a fertility preservation exercise.

In clinic, women without periods often want to do the Tonic, in which case I suggest that they follow the moon phase. The full moon is Day 1 and the new moon is Day 14. Even if you just Nourish from Days 1-14 and Warm from Days 14-28 you will still have some benefits.

The Menstrual Optimisation Plan (*see pages 46–58*) is ideal for women with a regular cycle. If your cycle is irregular you may find it becomes regular after following the Menstrual Tonic, or you may wish to subtly adapt the phases of the Optimisation Plan to suit your cycle.

The Body-Mind-Gut Programme

This programme (*see pages 72–80*) is great for anyone who has digestive issues. Over the years I have identified that many women (and men) suffer from digestive weakness and this is not separate from their reproductive system. Western medicine studies and practises all the different systems in the body in isolation: for example, the cardiologist studies at the heart, the gynaecologist studies the female reproductive system and there is not much attention given to the holistic overview of the body. In reality these systems are interdependent and overlapping. This is especially true of the reproductive and digestive systems. I would also recommend this chapter if you have been diagnosed as auto-immune or have immune system problems, a history of irritable bowel syndrome (IBS) or general digestive disturbance.

Fertile eggs

Improving egg quality is the holy grail of fertility treatment. I would recommend the chapter on fertile eggs (*see pages 85–92*) for women in their thirties and over wishing to optimise egg quality, or women preparing for IVF who want to increase their chances.

Miscarriage

The chapter on miscarriage (*see pages 93–100*) is for anyone who has a history of miscarriage.

Male fertility

For the very important man in your life, Fertile Man (*see pages 101–108*) explains how to optimise his fertility.

IVF support

In IVF Support (*see pages 109–120*) you will find information on how to prepare for and support yourself during IVF. The chapter includes a menu planner.

Don't panic

Not a week goes by without a story in the press about how women's fertility takes a huge nosedive in our mid- to late thirties. Yet the same papers and magazines simultaneously taunt us with images of celebrities who never age and seem to have babies well into their forties. It's often a matter of constitution, environment, lifestyle – and luck. Oh, and the man does have quite a bit to do with it!

The first thing to say is that yes, our fertility does indeed decline with age. However, while science will have it that we are all alike and will all decline at the same speed and age, this is not my experience.

Much of the data we have available regarding pregnancy rates in older women is taken from IVF clinics so it is likely that these women had fertility issues in the first place. That said, fertility does not last for ever, and older women will often have to make more dramatic changes to their lifestyles than younger women who have age on their side. DON'T PANIC and don't become obsessed. But DO take some steps now to optimise your fertility and general health to find out how fertile you are likely to be.

Fertility is a peripheral requirement for a human being. In other words, we don't need it in order to survive in the short term. So nature has a coping mechanism that, when our bodies are under stress or in danger, fertility is temporarily suspended. Of course, most of the people I see are not in immediate danger of being savaged by a tiger. Nevertheless, they are under stress in terms of their nervous and immune systems and often their digestive systems – in short, their systems are fighting constantly and it's a strain.

When we feel safe we release brain chemicals in a way that sends messages to the body that we are safe and that is an optimal time to conceive.

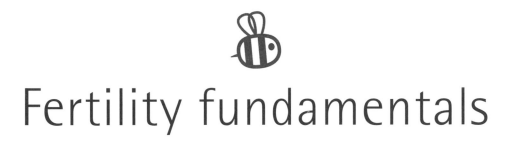

Fertility fundamentals

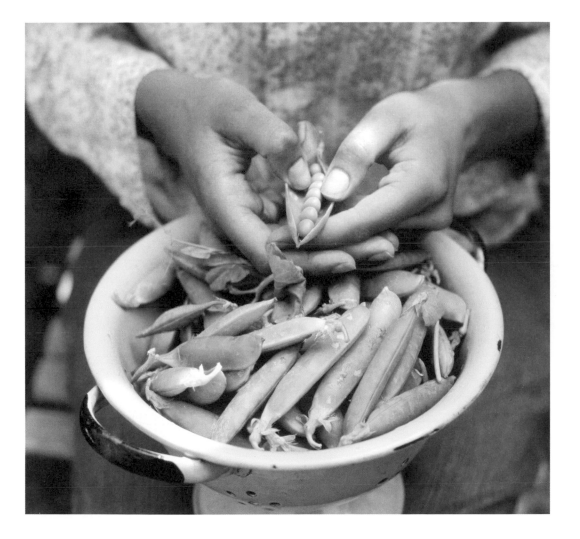

Our fertility is very precious and it does not last for ever. The way we choose to live our lives will inevitably affect our overall health and our fertility. Of course, there are factors in life that we are unable to change, for example, our inherited constitution, accidents and some illnesses. Lifestyle, however, is an area where those wishing to conceive can exert some control. This chapter outlines how lifestyle choices may impact on your fertility, how you can make wise choices to boost your chances of conceiving, and how other choices may negate fertility.

Fertile weight

Getting to the correct weight to have a baby can make a big difference to your chances. A fertile weight is neither too heavy nor too light. Of course, this does not mean that very thin women can't fall pregnant nor that women who are overweight will necessarily struggle; there are always exceptions to the rule. However, there is an optimum window that is considered to be healthy for conception.

What the research says

Increased weight is associated with reduced fertility in both sexes. There is a great deal of focus on women who are obese, but there is also a growing fertility issue with women who are too thin. There is now evidence to suggest that being either extremely over- or underweight may have a negative effect on fertility.[1]

Body fat helps convert the male hormone androgen into oestrogen. It's also been shown that having too little body fat can affect the menstrual cycle, and you may stop ovulating even if you are having periods each month. There is also a higher risk of miscarrying in the first trimester of pregnancy[2] – women with a low body mass index (BMI) are 72 per cent more likely to suffer a first trimester miscarriage.[3]

On the other hand, being overweight can affect your fertility too. You may develop insulin resistance, which can lead to an overproduction of the hormone leptin. This can contribute to irregular ovulation, or again an absence of ovulation altogether. Obese women suffer about eight more fetal and infant deaths per thousand births than women who enter pregnancy at a recommended weight.[3]

In IVF treatment, studies show that obese women are more likely to yield fewer follicles, fewer eggs are successfully collected and are of poorer quality, and implantation rates are lower, as are rates of pregnancy and live births.[4]

The distribution of fat is also significant. Excess lower body fat around the hips and bottom (pear-shaped) may affect fertility, but to a lesser extent than fat around the middle (apple-shaped).

The simplest way to check if your weight might be impacting on your fertility is to check your BMI. To do this, divide your weight in kilograms by your height in metres then divide the answer by your height again. (The NHS website has a handy online BMI calculator.) The optimum BMI for fertility is considered to be between 20 and 24, a slightly narrower range than for the general population, so if you are below or above you might want to take steps to lose or gain weight. The good news is that if you eat a healthy diet and take regular exercise, your body will naturally reach a healthy weight, unless you have a pre-existing condition that is affecting your weight, for example, a thyroid condition.

Preparation

You will need to put time aside to prioritise food and planning to make healthy meals. Plan your meals and make sure you have all the ingredients that you will need. This will help you to avoid reaching for the empty calories, skipping meals because there is nothing healthy or overeating the wrong food. I keep lots of useful ingredients to hand, like frozen chicken broth, herbs, nuts and seeds, so that I can always prepare a meal pretty quickly.

Portion size

It is important to feel sated from your meal or you will be tempted by unhealthy snacks. Eat just enough to satisfy yourself. It can be helpful to use the palm of your hand to measure portion sizes. Your fist is a good portion size for carbohydrates like wholegrains, and you can use the palm of your hand to measure the size of your protein source.

Healthy weight tips

- Don't cut back on good fats. Remember that good fats are a fertile food: avocado, oily fish, olive oils, coconut oil and nuts are all healthy (*see page 38*).
- Limit sugar in all its forms – even fruit needs to be kept to a minimum.
- Eat three meals a day and eat your last meal no later than 7pm. I am not a fan of snacking and believe the digestive system needs to rest and digest, particularly at night, which is why I advise people to stop eating early and let the system rest overnight. This is one of the best weight-loss methods I know; resting the digestion.
- Chew your food and be mindful of each mouthful (*see page 23*). Focus on the food and the nutrition you are receiving from it.
- Do not flood the system with water or other fluids. Drinking with food dilutes the digestive enzymes and weakens the 'digestive fire'.
- Feel grateful for the food on your plate and do not view it as the enemy. Think about how it got to your plate and choose foods that are as fertile as possible and not ones that have been mass-produced and therefore lack nutrients.

Balance

Many people decide to lose or gain weight and go on extreme diets. This is not sustainable and not preferable for fertility patients. If you lose weight too quickly the brain gets the signal that there are not enough calories available and that the body fat is dropping. On an evolutionary level this would have been a survival mechanism and it sends a signal that it isn't a good time to conceive as you may starve! It is always better to lose or gain weight gradually and in a balanced way. That way it is more likely to be a permanent change.

What, when and why of eating

For a long time now we have known that what we eat impacts on our health. It is also worth thinking about when you eat, as I believe regularity of foods and set meals is very important. Animal studies demonstrate that the time at which food is eaten, as well as the length of time left between meals, do have an impact on health.[5]

But perhaps even more important are the reasons behind why we eat. These can be complex and varied but people eat or don't eat for all different emotional reasons. It is important to address the emotional aspect to eating while trying to adjust your weight. Keep a journal and record your feelings. Do you reach for the chocolate when you feel insecure or sad? Do you regularly skip meals and avoid food as a way of gaining control in your life? Do you eat mindlessly, not engaging in the food? It is important to be really honest about your relationship with food. It is such a fundamental building block for our health and fertility, yet it has for many become a battlefield for unmet emotional needs.

If you need help with these issues, Overeaters Anonymous runs a programme of recovery for eating issues, including compulsive eating, overeating, undereating, obesity, anorexia and bulimia.

Low self-esteem

Low self-esteem can play havoc with all our plans and sabotage even the best intentions. We all go through feelings of doubt and not feeling good enough. I call it 'coming from a place of lack'. There will never be enough food, money, babies, happiness, men or jobs to go around. This can leave us with a desperately empty feeling, particularly when we want something badly and it isn't happening. Try to be kind to yourself. Part of being fertile is living with abundant thinking (not lack thinking); try to change your thought process towards there always being enough of everything to go round. Think of all the great things about yourself and your life and bring that feeling into your being.

Eating disorders

Anorexia, bulimia and orthorexia (being obsessed with eating healthily) are all prevalent among women (and increasingly men); they result from, and result in, severe disruption in the body/mind system. They are the ultimate act in denying yourself nourishment and nutrition. On an emotional and spiritual level, when we deny the body such a basic need we are actually destroying and sabotaging ourselves; it is the ultimate act of self-destruction. Our ability to receive nourishment and love is exactly the ability we need to develop in order to receive a child into our being.

If you are struggling with an eating disorder it is imperative that you seek help. Over the years I have treated countless women who struggle with their weight, on the one hand wanting a baby, on the other wishing to remain thin. It is a deep conflict within women that can cause irreversible damage within their systems. It leads to hormonal imbalance, lack of nutrients, heart weakness and deep-rooted emotional issues.

Exercise

Modern exercise trends, which include 'boot-camp'-style workouts, Bikram ('hot') yoga and triathlons tend to be extreme and not conducive to conceiving. Many people are running on empty and depleted in vital energy. In some people, the body may not have enough energy to support both intense physical training and pregnancy.[6] For example, more than three hours of aerobic exercise a day has been shown to reduce pregnancy rates in IVF patients.[7] However, regular and moderate exercise has been shown to improve blood flow and reduce oxidative stress, which may improve fertility.[8] Women who have a high BMI see improvements in their fertility with moderate exercise.[7] But prolonged vigorous cycling (more than five hours in one session) has been shown to adversely affect sperm.[7]

My view is that vigorous exercise can deplete the vital substances – the Qi (vital energy), the Blood and ultimately the Jing. But when practised appropriately, mindful exercises – such as yoga, meditation, walking, dancing, cycling (although not so great for sperm), rebound exercise and anything that creates movement but not exhaustion – cultivate Qi and therefore are likely to benefit fertility. Moderate exercise moves Qi and calms the emotions.

Taking exercise is an important aspect of living a fertile life. However, many people now either exercise too little or too much. Of course, levels of exercise are entirely individual and we must all find our perfect level. It is important that you find something you enjoy and that it does not feel like a chore. Try to pick an exercise that you love. Research shows that if exercise has a social element it increases its effectiveness.

If you need to lose weight exercise may be an important aspect of this. It is still important to take it slowly and don't launch into a programme that is exhausting and depleting. If the body is adrenally stressed and exhausted it will hold on to the weight.

Running

Running is of particular note, such is its rise in popularity. In the 1970s running was actually considered to be bad for you by some people. I am afraid that I have to reinforce this message. I am not one to take things that help them feel better away from people, and of course many people around

Exercise guidelines

- If you are just starting out – take it slowly and gradually build it up.
- Do not exercise when exhausted or ill.
- Do not exercise after heavy blood loss.
- Twenty minutes of movement every day will bring health benefits.
- Do not exercise in over-heated rooms – excessive sweating depletes our energy. People with excessive Dampness (*see page 31*) are the only exception to this as they can afford to lose excessive fluids.
- Do exercise you enjoy.

the world have benefitted from running – a little. But for women wanting to conceive I believe there are better ways to keep fit. In our evolution there would have been two types of situation in which we would have run. In the first type we were chasing something to eat because we were starving hungry, and in the second we were running for our life as we were being chased by something else that was starving hungry! In both situations our bodies would produce high levels of adrenaline to give us the energy to perform this extra feat to ensure our survival. And that is just it: on an evolutionary level running was something we did to survive. Adrenaline sends the message to our brains that we are in danger. This is not the optimal condition for conception.

There will be many people who conceive while running, even training for marathons. We are all different, but my observation is that in women who are struggling to conceive, those who over-exercise, particularly those who run, often do better from reducing or stopping running. If you are running to reduce stress, you are probably just putting your body under a different kind of stress. It might be helpful to find other ways to relieve stress. Acupuncture works really well, as do dancing, singing or walking in nature.

Digestion

My mantra is: diet is important but digestion is everything. I see many fertility patients and women with irregular menstrual cycles who have compromised digestion – it's very common.

- To improve digestion, preferably only eat raw foods in the morning and not after 4pm.
- Irregular eating and eating when stressed or upset all injure digestion. It is important to eat regularly, give time to food and eat while relaxed.

- Bloating may indicate that your digestion is too weak to process raw food in the evening, which is when your digestion begins to slow down naturally. Instead of raw leaves for salads, eat warm salads made with lightly steamed or roasted vegetables in the evenings.
- Skipping meals can also be a cause of bloating.
- Chew your food slowly to aid digestion. It is the first step in the chemical and physical digestion of your food. Chewing for longer helps you absorb more nutrients from your food, maintain a healthy weight and leads to fewer digestive problems, such as bloating and gas. How many times you should chew depends on what you are eating; chew until your mouthful of food has lost all of its texture.
- Eat as early as you are able in the evening to give your body longer to digest your food.
- Broth is nourishing and nutrient-dense, full of amino acids and minerals as well as collagen and cartilage. It has a long reputation as a healing food and it may help with inflammation and digestive problems. You can use broth as a drink and in soups, stews and to cook wholegrains and rice.

Stress

Stress is all around us; my observation is that in the past ten years we have become more stressed and more tired than previous generations, despite all our marvellous time-saving devices! Research studies demonstrate that the likelihood of becoming pregnant is reduced when stress levels are high.[9] A recent American study of 501 couples over 12 months found a 29 per cent reduction in fertility and a two-fold increase in risk of infertility in couples demonstrating high levels of stress.[10]

There are many ways that stress can become an issue in our lives. Some of these are out of our control, but many are within our control. Some of the stress we experience is what I term 'stress of our own making'. In other words, we create or attract stress in our life by our own actions, thought processes or by our unconscious behaviour.

In clinic I observe that patients who become obsessed with their fertility tend to be less happy, engage less socially and have reduced libido. The higher the stress levels are, the longer it takes couples to conceive and the higher their levels of stress rise[11]. I want to encourage you to develop self-awareness rather than being ultra-vigilant, which creates rigidity.

Lowering stress levels brings many benefits to couples trying to conceive. It is really important for you to find ways to live a calmer life. Sometimes it is simply a matter of acknowledging how much noise there is in your mind and deciding to switch off. Women often get worried after one month of trying that there is something wrong. It is completely normal for it to take several months to get pregnant; it is perfectly normal for it to take up to a year. Most couples are not infertile, but subfertile, so improving your diet and lifestyle and living a more fertile life will improve the chances every month of conceiving. Stressing about how long it is taking will not help anything.

Many couples I see are impatient and not infertile. We are so used to getting what we want by working harder and doing, it can be hard to accept that things are not always within our control.

The more out of control we feel, the more controlling we become. It is a vicious cycle. I always say, 'What is so good about control anyway? All the best things happen when we let go of control – like LOVE, for example.'

Overwork

Overwork is a growing problem in society and will likely continue to impact both male and female health and fertility. The effects of overwork on fertility are not well covered by current research, although I see it as a huge problem and one that shows no sign of abating. Working long hours without taking adequate rest, the pressure of moving up the career ladder, over-exercising at the end of a long day, over-communication, social media, smart phones, using computers before bed, not recuperating after illness, miscarriage; all these and more take their toll on our bodies and on our energy systems. In order to preserve and optimise fertility it is vital to take adequate rest and not to exhaust your energy.

Protect yourself from STDs

Sexually transmitted diseases (STDs) are the most common cause of fallopian tube disorders, which make up about 20 per cent of female infertility. Chlamydia can lie completely undetected with no

Fertile womb breathing exercise

This exercise will help you calm a monkey mind. Do it whenever you find that you are over-thinking. It will help you become more aware of how much time you spend thinking and worrying about things that have not happened, may never happen and over which you are powerless.

1 Lie or sit and be comfortable.

2 Place your hands, palms down, on your lower abdomen, below your tummy button and above your pubic bone.

3 Shut your eyes and breathe deeply, inhaling through your nose and out through a small opening between your lips.

4 Feel your abdomen rise and fall. It is almost impossible to be in your mind when you do this. Let your thoughts pass like clouds in the sky. Breathe and let go.

symptoms and result in blocked fallopian tubes if not diagnosed and treated early on. It is important to use barrier methods of contraception, such as condoms, until you are with a partner who you might want to have children with. This is the best way to protect you from STDs.

Regular tests will mean that if you have contracted anything then you can get early treatment, which might help prevent a condition from developing into something more serious and harder to treat.

Alcohol

Drinking as little as two units per day can have a negative impact on female fertility and excessive alcohol consumption has been found to cause infertility.[12] The negative effects of excessive alcohol consumption on fertility include increased time to conception, anovulation (no ovulation), luteal phase dysfunction, poor or abnormal embryo development and even early menopause.[13] Evidence regarding 'safe' levels of alcohol intake in terms of fertility is not conclusive and it is often confusing trying to work out how much is safe or if you should be drinking at all.

The evidence for occasional alcohol consumption is less clear than that for excessive drinking: in a Danish study women who drank alcohol moderately (two glasses per week) conceived more quickly than women who drank no alcohol[14]. A study looking at 7,760 women found no negative effects from alcohol on fertility in younger women, although in the same study women over 30 who consumed more than seven alcoholic drinks per week were more likely to experience infertility than women who drank less than one per week.[15]

Like so many of these things, it is likely that moderation is the best route, but moderation really is quite moderate, and some people find it easier not to drink at all. Alcohol can become a bone of contention between couples, creating resentment if one partner abstains while the other does not. For women with poor egg quality and men with poor sperm results, I suggest abstinence. The National Institute for Health and Care Excellence (NICE) and the Royal College of Obstetricians and Gynaecologists (RCOG) state that women trying to conceive should avoid alcohol altogether.

Alcohol affects people in different ways and some people are definitely more adversely affected than others. As women age their ability to process alcohol reduces and this may well be why research shows that alcohol has a more negative effect on older women. The self-assessment in the next chapter (*see pages 28–37*) is useful with regards to who may be most likely to be negatively affected by drinking. Those who present with too much Heat or too much Damp often are much better off avoiding alcohol. A small amount of alcohol can help to move Stagnation and calm the mind.

Smoking

Research consistently demonstrates that smoking negatively impacts both male and female fertility.[16] Smoking increases the risks of miscarriage and ectopic pregnancy, adversely impacts semen quality and sperm count, and reduces the chances of IVF success.[17] Women whose mothers smoked during

Ten ways to live a fertile life

1 Honour your body.
2 Keep a calm mind – have a digital curfew once a week and a daily screen-time limit.
3 Eat real food.
4 Get adequate rest; do not overwork or over-exercise.
5 Know thyself: address your issues.
6 Make time for sex and become a better lover.
7 Remember that acceptance and gratitude are healing forces in our life.
8 Don't compare yourself to others.
9 Respect your community and environment.
10 Shift your mind from doing to being and receiving.

pregnancy had a reduction in their egg quality.[18] And other research demonstrates that women who smoked during assisted reproductive treatment (ART) were less likely to become pregnant or have a live birth, and were more likely to have an ectopic pregnancy or miscarry.[19]

My observations over many years tell me that women with a history of smoking are likely to have depleted their fertile fluids – their 'Yin fluids'. In my experience, women who are Yin deficient struggle to produce good quality embryos. Smoking will make this situation even worse. From a reproductive point of view it is the single worse thing you can do to your fertility.

Recreational drugs

Recreational drugs can cause subfertility in both men and women.[20] Women who smoke marijuana are more likely to experience primary infertility than non-users.[21] Smoking marijuana may delay ovulation and negatively impact on embryo development.[22] In men, marijuana has a negative impact on sperm, and may also prevent sperm from being able to fertilise an egg.[23]

Although in the short term cocaine can improve sexual performance, long-term users report a decrease in sexual function, including difficulties in maintaining an erection and ejaculating.[24] Patients with a history of drug use often stop in their bid to conceive. As with any substance misuse, the harm done will depend on individual constitution and the type and extent of drugs used. Those with a background of recreational drug used frequently show signs of Yin deficiency, too much heat in the liver, Qi stagnation, Jing deficiency and even emotional problems.

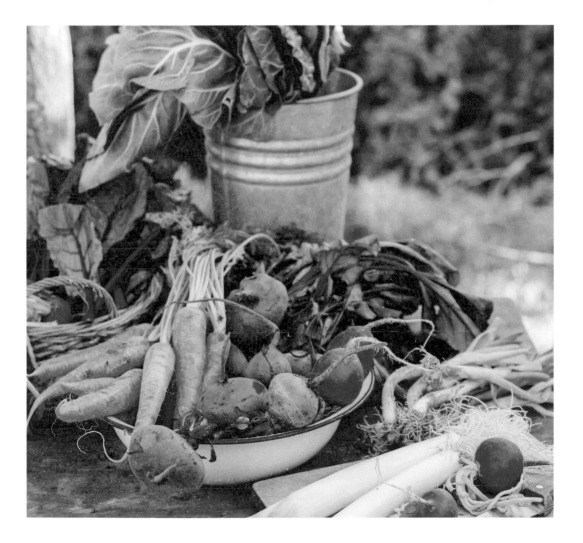

Fertile food

Eating well and cooking delicious food is a fertile and healthy activity to be celebrated. Unfortunately, many women (and increasingly men) without realising subscribe to diets that may be detrimental to good health and fertility, cutting out grains or fats that are essential to our hormonal balance.

Don't obsess about food

Many women place too much control around food, which results in food becoming an issue. Rigidity is not healthy, especially in our attitude to eating. Ultimately it creates another tension in the body and the digestion and can lead to a deepening of the issue with food.

A fertile diet is abundant in nature's miracles. It is seasonal, colourful, varied, mindful and plentiful. It warms us when we feel cold, cools when we are hot and bothered, gets our energy flowing when we feel stuck and addresses any imbalances we may be feeling.

Sceptics will say, 'Oh yeah, sure! If I eat more beans I'm going to get pregnant!' This is not what I am saying, nor is it the premise of the book or my approach to fertility. However, food and digestion are the building blocks for good health and, along with the rest of the lifestyle choices we make, it is the one area where we are able to make healthy and fertile decisions.

Many of you will be fascinated to discover the connection between our emotions, how we eat, what we eat and how we feel. In China there are restaurants that ask you how you feel today and then bring you appropriate dishes to balance your condition; such is the relationship between food and health. I have seen so often in my clinic how choosing food that heals us rather than harms us is part of living a more fertile life.

Our diet can be a way of life that supports our health, rather than a regime. Even the simple enjoyment of food increases its nourishment as our body finds it easier to digest food when we are relaxed. When we eat a meal that is balanced, we gain more from the meal as a whole than from the separate parts. When we share food we are happier, and the same goes for when we create rituals around food such as lighting candles, having flowers on the table and presenting the food in visually appealing ways. Romance is good for our health and our fertility. This is the approach that I use with patients, treating them as a whole person whose emotions and lifestyle all form part of the picture even if they have come to me with a specific condition.

Balancing your fertile tendencies

Part of what I do with patients is to help improve the way the body functions and what I often refer to as their 'energetic tendencies' or 'internal climate'. This is about making the soil (the body) more balanced and therefore more fertile. We all have a leaning towards a particular constitution that means when we are out of balance we will be likely to experience certain symptoms or tendencies.

The internal climates can be categorised as: Cold, Damp, Blood Deficient (dryness), Hot, Stagnant, Blood Stagnant. This may sound a little alien at first but actually it is very instinctual. We all recognise

Our busy, busy lives

Many people complain to me that they are far too busy to buy and prepare healthy foods. Of course, preparing home-made food often does take longer than opening a ready-made meal, but healthy food does not have to be more expensive or take twice the time to prepare. It is often more a question of being organised and making food a priority. People also say to me that they do not have enough time for making love. I think we all need to be honest about what our priorities are and it is up to us as individuals to re-evaluate how we spend our time. When you eat well you will have more time and more energy because you will be ill less often and feel great.

For me, living a more fertile life means slowing down and making time for the things that feed my soul. Making time for food, making time to 'smell the roses', making time for laughter, loved ones, taking someone who has just had a hard time a home-made meal. For you it might be a very different list; this is not a 'things I have to do' list, a list of 'shoulds' and 'oughts'; this is a 'things that make my heart sing' list.

It's amazing when you ask people what they consider important – it's nearly always the small things. When I talk to groups of women, I talk about how we have given up many things that matter. How, for all the time-saving devices we have, we actually have less time and do fewer of the things in life that connect us to our fellow human beings. We have less intimacy, less connection, less family time and we are lonelier, more addicted, more in debt, more overweight, less fertile and more isolated than ever. The choice is ours; unless we want to lose the things we value forever we need to take small steps to reclaim what we are losing. It starts with you!

if we are someone who feels the cold or burns up easily, but we may be less familiar with concepts such as Dampness or Stagnation. It is interesting and fun to discover a little more about our tendencies; the important thing is not to get fixated on being just one. Most of us are a lovely mixture of all these and that makes us well balanced. What is interesting about the process of understanding the climates is it helps us develop self-awareness and self-knowledge.

Bringing our body back into a natural balance is one of the most powerful ways to nourish our fertility and wellbeing. Terms like Hot and Cold may sound simplistic, but actually improving our internal climate can have a profound impact on our fertility.

Cold tendency

You may have always been too Cold, or you may have pushed your constitution in the direction of Cold by consuming too many cold, raw foods. I typically see this in women who have dieted on juices, raw foods and salads. Sometimes the body can become too Cold from medication (antibiotics are very Cold in nature). Or Cold can penetrate externally when spending too much time outside in the elements or (for people who work in supermarkets) being blown on by cold air pumping out from the fridges.

Traditionally in Chinese culture a womb that was too Cold was said to be the major cause of infertility. This still holds partly true today, although as the planet has become hotter so have we and I think this is changing. What I do see a lot of is Cold impacting on sexual function and menstrual cycles – Cold tends to make things move more slowly and leads to Stagnation. The effect on the menstrual cycle is that the periods are often delayed and painful and made better through heat.

Think of this tendency as an icy pond. Nothing much will thrive here as it is just too cold and lacking in movement.

Symptom checklist

- You have an abdomen that is cold to touch.
- You have water retention.
- You sometimes have menstrual pain – which improves with heat application.
- You have abdominal pain that is worse for pressure.
- The colour of the period is dark purple.
- You have a white coat on your tongue.
- You have a pale complexion.
- You have a sluggish digestion.
- Your urine is pale.
- You may have a longer menstrual cycle.
- You put on weight easily.
- You have a medium to low libido.
- You would rather stay in with a good book and a hot water bottle.

Warming foods and remedies

- Warming foods include: almonds, beetroot, carrots, cayenne pepper, chicken, chocolate, cinnamon, cloves, figs, garlic, ginger, lamb, mustard, nutmeg, peaches, peppers, pumpkin, radishes, sesame seeds, squash, tomatoes (cooked).
- Add cinnamon, ginger, cardamom, garlic and clove to food.
- Eating cooked foods is preferable to raw foods, which are cold in nature and will make the body colder. Steamed and sautéed vegetables with added spices are ideal.
- If eating fruit, cooking it with spices will improve the warming function.
- Eat salads in moderation and early in the day.
- Avoid oranges, mangoes, pineapples and grapes, all of which cool the body further.
- Try a dukkah mix (*see page 168*) with cayenne, ginger, pepper, chestnut, pistachio or walnut.
- Warming teas: chai, ginger.

Damp tendency

This is common with people who live in humid climates or people who work in damp or humid places. Chefs sometimes suffer from Dampness as they have to work where there is a lot of vapour. I have also seen people who live in basement flats suffer from Dampness. People who consume a lot of dairy, or excessive amounts of sweet or greasy fried goods tend to accumulate Dampness. Or you may have a reasonable diet but a poor digestion and the food does not digest properly so Dampness accumulates in the system. There is a lack of transformation and this leads to Dampness and Stagnation.

Think of this tendency as a dark, dank pool of water that is starting to fester.

Symptom checklist

- You suffer from allergies or skin conditions.
- You may suffer from candida or thrush.
- You have cellulite.
- You are sedentary.
- You 'crash out' when you go to sleep.
- Your body feels heavy.
- You find it difficult to concentrate and you have a fuzzy head.
- You have a sticky taste in the mouth.
- You may have a stuffy chest.

Damp-resolving foods and remedies

- Damp-resolving foods include: aduki beans, alfalfa sprouts (avoid all sprouts when pregnant), asparagus, barley, basil, buckwheat, caraway, cardamom, celery, coriander, corn, endives, horseradish, lemons, parsley.
- Garlic, horseradish, kohlrabi and mustard greens are all pungent and help with Damp conditions.
- Barley water is an excellent remedy. Add barley and parsley to food.
- It is important for you not to be eating too much food, especially in the evening. Try not to make your meals too complex and chew your food very well.
- Avoid sugar, bread, pasta, beer, orange juice and tomato pastes and purées.
- Too many nuts may also make your condition worse, although seeds are fine, so opt for sesame seeds, pumpkin seeds, sunflower seeds. Of the nuts, walnut and almond are best tolerated.
- Reduce wheat.
- Move more – stretching is especially good.
- You would do very well on the Body-Mind-Gut Programme (*see pages 72–80*).
- Damp-resolving teas: green, jasmine (drink with meals).

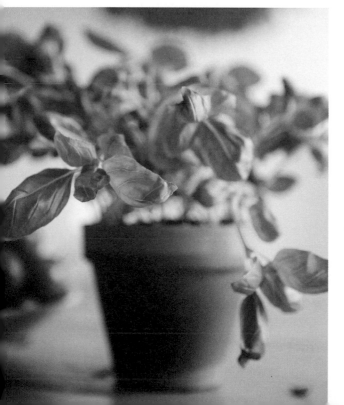

The mind and Dampness

There is often a psychological aspect to Dampness and it can be helpful to look at our shadow self. Where have we been wounded in the past and how does this impact on us in the present time? All of our responses come from a previous wound or shadow, which can play out throughout our life. Perhaps we have a deep-seated fear of rejection or inadequacy that creates an emotional heaviness to our personality. Taking responsibility for how we are in the world and 'owning our stuff' can be very healing. Lightening up emotionally and having fun is a good antidote to Dampness and heaviness.

Nettles

Nettles are one of nature's great gifts to man; granted, they do sting a little when you touch them but they are full of goodness and easily available.

Nettles are a particular favourite of mine because of their Blood-nourishing qualities. They are also full of vitamin C and a great anti-inflammatory. There is a tree that comes out in my garden in early Spring, a variety of birch. I am so allergic to it and it gives me the most terrible streaming eyes and nose. But every year I find that if I remember to dose myself up with nettle tea for a few weeks before it comes out and continue while it is out my symptoms are really reduced.

Drink nettle tea post period in the NOURISH phase (*see page 48*).

Blood Deficient tendency

Many women present with Blood Deficient symptoms, normally after their period. Even if you don't fully identify with this pattern, I often encourage women to nourish their blood on days 7—13 of their cycle. The blood in our body is mostly made through the food we eat and the air we breathe. But a good digestion is also important.

Many women today run on empty, overdo it, skip meals, over-exercise or exercise when tired or in over-heated rooms and don't take adequate rest. Typically a woman who is constantly on the go and on a diet will be Blood Deficient. A person with strong blood will have plentiful, shiny hair and a healthy complexion. Dry skin and hair and cracking nails are a sure sign the blood is weak. You have scant periods. Blood deficiency can also occur literally after losing a lot of blood, breast-feeding too long (this is an individual thing) or from suffering an emotional shock or trauma that injures the spirit and depletes the blood.

Think of this as the vampire tendency – pale and weak without sufficient supplies of blood.

Symptom checklist

- You have dry, dull skin and hair.
- Your lips and tongue are pale.
- Your nails are dry and brittle.
- You are often forgetful.
- You may suffer from dizziness and/or little dots or floaters in your vision.
- You may find it difficult to fall asleep and have vivid dreams (this means the heart's blood is weak).
- You tend to push yourself and don't rest enough.
- You feel anxious.
- Your mind is restless.
- You may have a slim build.

Blood-nourishing foods and remedies

- Blood-nourishing foods include: aduki beans, apricots, beef, beetroot, bone marrow, cherries, dandelions, dates, eggs, figs, grapes, kale, kidney beans, leafy greens, meat, mussels, nettles, octopus, oysters, parsley, sardines, seaweed, squid, sweet rice, tempeh, watercress.
- Green chlorophyll-rich foods, such as spinach, parsley, broccoli, asparagus and wheatgrass, are very good for nourishing blood.
- Protein-rich foods are also very important. Include lots of dark foods in the diet: black and red beans (well soaked), black and red fruits, black sesame seeds.
- Make a super seed mix or dukkah (*see page 168*) to sprinkle on foods, salads, porridge, vegetables.
- Avoiding sugar is important as it 'consumes the blood' and causes an imbalance.
- Alcohol is a problem for Blood Deficient types as it tends to be heating and therefore dries the blood.
- Rest is very important and it is vital not to over-exercise. Obsessive exercise is fast becoming a problem in our obsessive culture. Only moderate exercise is advised for Blood Deficient types who may well need to reduce their exercise down to 15-20 minutes of moderate exercise per day (with two days' rest every week in order for their blood deficiency to improve).
- Blood-nourishing teas: nettle.

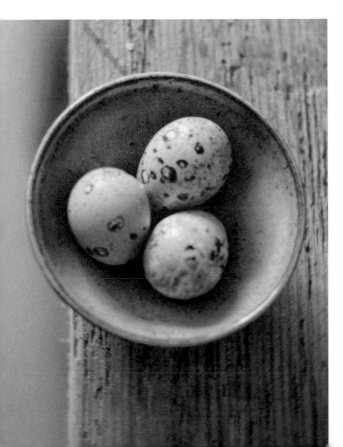

Hot tendency

The body needs to be warm to function properly – the problem is that when it gets too hot the body becomes inflamed. This is a growing issue and I suspect that as the earth gets hotter, so do we.

Heat comes about in the system through unreleased and pent-up emotions, from exposure to too many toxins internally and externally, and through eating or drinking too many Heating foods and substances. Drugs also Heat the body, and working-out and dancing in very hot rooms while drinking alcohol and/or taking drugs really Heats the body.

Think of this tendency as the pressure cooker – the heat is building up and you are going to explode if you don't let off steam or cool down.

When our bodies have too much Heat they are prone to inflammation, our minds stress out and our heart feels agitated.

It is very important to be mindful about where in your life you are generating Heat. Is it emotional from being pent-up and unable to express your emotions or are you over-indulging in too many Heating substances? If the cause is emotional, then attempting to bring the body back into balance through food alone will only go so far. You will need to do some soul-searching and look for the emotional causes and take steps to address these. Bringing relaxation into your life and doing activities that help you to switch off will literally help you cool down; 'chill out, man'.

Symptom checklist

- You often feel thirsty.
- You throw the covers off the bed at night.
- You feel 'charged'.
- You have a temper and react strongly to things.
- You are often agitated and find it difficult to relax.
- You have periods that come earlier than expected or are heavy.
- You are prone to fevers and inflammation.
- Your periods are very red in colour.

Cooling foods and remedies

- Cooling foods include: apples, aubergines, bitter salad leaves, cottage cheese, crab, cress, cucumbers, grapefruit, lemons, lettuce, mung bean soup, mussels, pork, pears, milk (cow's or soya), spinach, tofu, tomatoes (raw), yoghurt.
- This is the one condition that responds well to raw foods so adding a raw element to a meal can help a lot.
- Bitter and sour-tasting foods are also important; chicory is ideal. Grated vegetables in a sauce as a condiment to a meal are very helpful, as is a side of salad or steamed vegetables. Teacher and author Daverick Leggett recommends grated white radish with a splash of soya sauce.
- Cooling teas: green, mint, peppermint, rose.

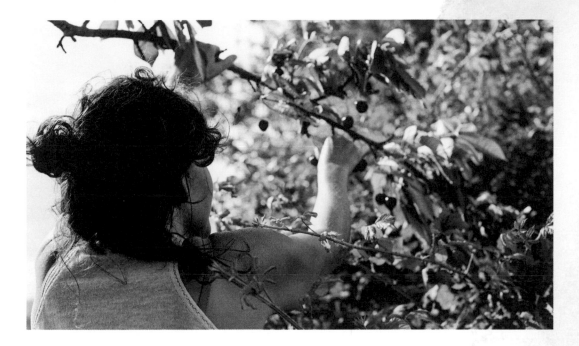

Stagnant (Qi) tendency

We become Stagnant when our plans are thwarted and when we can't get to where we want to be. When we are living out of balance with our true nature, we become stuck and frustrated and cannot see the wood for the trees. Stagnation leads to depression and it is common in modern society because the way we are living is so alien to our true nature – which is to be free and to be creative. No wonder there is so much depression when we are not living in harmony with the natural rhythm of life and we have become totally disconnected from our environment and nature. No wonder we have become less fertile.

So much of fertility has to do with movement and flow; the egg is released each month and it must travel down the fallopian tubes in order to meet with the sperm, which must also make its hard journey through the cervix. The fertilised egg must then find a place to implant on the uterus wall where it will be nourished through a regular flow of blood. All of this requires a good flow of Qi, but many couples suffer from Stagnation of energy, as a result of sedentary lives or through being emotionally frustrated. This pattern is very common in couples who have been trying to conceive for a while.

On a physical level Stagnation disrupts the digestion, causing pain and discomfort particularly in the epigastric (ribcage) area. Stagnation also disrupts the rhythm of the menstrual cycle. Irregularity of any kind is always a sign of Stagnation.

Symptom checklist

- You sigh a lot.
- You're indecisive or frustrated.
- You frown a lot.
- You have random aches in your body.
- You feel discomfort after eating.
- Your breasts often feel swollen or tender.
- Your periods are irregular.
- You find you belch.
- You have a history of IBS or other digestive complaints that often worsen when stressed.
- You feel 'stuck' and lacking in energy or vitality.

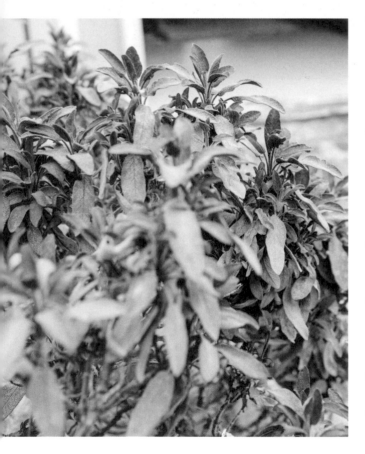

Moving foods and remedies

- Moving foods include: aubergines, beef, cherries, chestnuts, chilli, chives, coconut, cold water fish (sardines, mackerel), eggs, kohlrabi, leeks, lentils, molasses, oats, quinoa, sage, shiitake mushrooms, venison, saffron, sticky rice, turmeric, vinegar.
- Pickles served as a condiment are highly recommended, and carrots made into a soup with cumin, ginger or coriander are a perfect remedy for Stagnation.
- Add lemon peel to dishes as they are cooking and drink warm water and lemon or cider vinegar on rising.
- You need to get moving and exercise. You also need to get moving on an emotional front and be honest about the places in your life where you are stuck. It is time to change the story: join a club, go dancing, take responsibility for what is not working in your life.
- Talking therapy may help some people but for others it can keep them stuck even more in their story and actually make things worse. Building on your resources is very helpful for those who find talking does not help. Find what makes you happy and focus on that – do more of it.
- Gratitude is also really important; learn to focus on what you have in your life and what you are trying to create.
- Take up a new creative hobby and see it through. Set yourself targets and if you get stuck, find solutions or ask people for help and don't give up in frustration.
- You would do well on the Body-Mind-Gut Programme (*see pages 72–80*).
- Moving teas: Chamomile, fennel, jasmine, orange peel (with a meal).

Blood Stagnant tendency

Blood Stagnation is a step on from general (or Qi) Stagnation and it sometimes involves Cold as well. It can also occur after surgery or injury when the body has suffered physical trauma and the blood cannot move freely around the point of injury. Endometriosis and fibroids come under this category.

Think of this tendency as dark pools of blood collecting in the wrong places.

It is important not to let this condition go on for a long time if it is severe, as in the case of endometriosis or fibroids, you may need surgery to address the problem. Of course, surgery can cause more Stagnation so it is a fine balance, and appropriate medical advice is essential. This condition does respond well to treatment with acupuncture, and dietary changes can help too, but it really is a question of severity. I have had many patients over the years whose symptoms have improved thanks to changes in the diet and/or acupuncture. Equally, others have needed medical intervention to remove the physical Blood Stagnation that may be manifesting as fibroids or cysts.

One way I assess how severe the Stagnation has become is by looking underneath the tongue and looking for sublingual veins. If swollen, engorged and purple, the Stagnation is bad. Dark purple, black or red prickles on the tongue are also a good indicator. Spider veins on the tops of the thighs also tell me how well the blood is moving around the body. If the veins on the tops of the legs are visible it tells me the veins are under pressure and the blood is showing signs of Stagnating.

Symptom checklist

- You have fixed pain that is stabbing in nature.
- You have cysts.
- You have endometriosis.
- You have fibroids.
- You have fixed pain with your periods.
- You have clots in the menstrual blood.
- Your menstrual blood is dark or purple.
- You may suffer from headaches that are fixed and stabbing.

Moving foods and remedies

- Follow the advice for moving foods opposite but also include: butter, crab, onion, rose tea, spring onion, turnip, vinegar.
- Smoking hardens the arteries so if you are still smoking – stop!
- Massaging the limbs with a mixture of lavender and cypress oil diluted in a carrier helps to circulate the blood more effectively around the body.

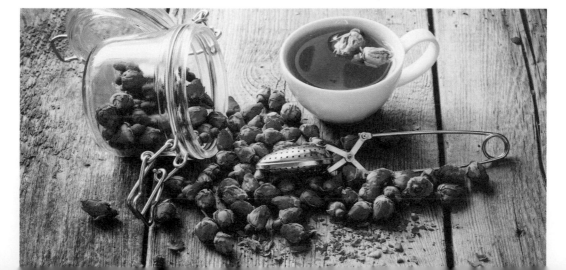

Healthy fats

Our bodies need essential fatty acids from the diet. These are vital to support immune function, healthy hormonal balance and to control inflammation in the body. Healthy fats from food such as oily fish, nuts (especially walnuts), seeds and avocados increase the production of anti-inflammatory prostaglandins and reduce the formation of pro-inflammatory ones. Prostaglandins regulate the female reproductive system and are involved in the control of ovulation and the menstrual cycle.

Fats have had a bad press for years but at last people are coming around to understanding that not all fat is bad for us. Using low-fat foods is a mistake as they not only rob us of essential fats but are often laced with other unhealthy substances to make them palatable. Eat food as near to its natural state as possible.

Essential fatty acids omega-3 and omega-6 (non-saturated fats) are what you are after. However, diets that are high in processed, unnatural foods and low in plant foods and oily fish tend to have too high a ratio of omega-6 to omega-3. Some experts believe this may be the reason why we suffer from so many problems that have their roots in chronic inflammation. Avoiding eating too many processed foods and eating plenty of oily fish (*see page 40*) will help you achieve the right balance (the ideal ratio of omega-6 to omega-3 is 4:1).

I use cold-pressed oils at home, such as olive and hemp oil. It is worth buying the best you can afford. These oils are very sensitive to light and heat and should be stored in a cool place and used up quite quickly once opened. Always buy them in dark, glass bottles and check they have been cold-pressed. Do not cook with these oils; instead, drizzle over cooked food or make into dressings for salads.

Cook with second-pressed or hot-pressed oil. Second-pressed olive oil tends to be cheaper than cold-pressed olive oil and is not stored in a dark bottle. Coconut oil and animal fats such as goose fat (or dripping) are stable at high temperatures and can also be used for cooking. Ghee is also great for cooking and is used in Indian cooking.

Butter can be used like cold-pressed oils; it can be melted but not heated to a high temperature. You can use it to lightly coat vegetables, sweat onions, make sauces, and so on. I like to add a flavoured butter like anchovy or garlic to meat after cooking. Do not buy the softened versions.

Dairy

Too much dairy in the diet can be quite Dampening. When consumed by someone who is already prone to Damp conditions, excess dairy can have a negative impact. Dampness in the body can affect the release of an egg at ovulation and also inhibit the passage through the fallopian tubes. It can also aggravate Damp-type allergies (so where there is a lot of phlegm involved) and make Damp and swollen-type joint pain worse.

It is also advisable to separate consumption of dairy from meat because the acids produced in the stomach to digest meat are neutralised by milk leading, to more Dampness.

Seasonal eating

The more we engage in the cycles and rhythms of the year and the natural world, the healthier and more fertile we are. Nature has so much to offer and if we returned to a time when we allowed ourselves to be more influenced by it then I am convinced we would be healthier. For example, if we went to bed earlier in the Winter and spent more time in reflective practice we would replenish our depleted energy supplies. If we picked and ate strawberries in the Summer instead of having them flown in from around the world at other times we would nourish ourselves and do less damage to the environment. The media encourage us to eat lots of particular so-called 'superfoods'. Often these foods are not indigenous to our country where perfectly nourishing foods already exist. Try to source about 60-70 per cent of your food locally and seasonally.

Some dairy is recommended, however (*see Nurses' Study, page 79*). Full-fat milk is preferable to skimmed or semi-skimmed, and warming milk with cardamom will make it easier to digest. My Chinese medicine colleague, author Daverick Leggett, explains: ' The removal of fat to make low-fat milk is probably misguided. Removing the fat imbalances the food and increases the chances of an adverse reaction in the body. When the level of fat is reduced the level of protein is relatively increased, which in turn overtaxes the kidneys'.

If someone has a genuine intolerance then consuming dairy will affect the immune system and will aggravate allergies and make the body more inflamed, causing more pain in those with painful conditions. In terms of fertility, too much inflammation may make the body less receptive and prevent implantation. That said, a small amount of good quality dairy products (full-fat, organic) can be tolerated by many women. Women who are lacking in moisture and tend to be dry can often benefit from a small amount of good quality organic milk (because it's a Yin tonic) as long as they have a strong digestion.

Juicing

I am not a fan of the juicing fad, especially for fertility. It is so often done by people who skip meals and wish to make up for it by consuming food in liquid form.

I would classify juice as 'overly nutritious'; cold, concentrated liquid entering the digestive system without having been chewed! In most people this injures the digestion and in the long term does not improve nutritional status.

As food is chewed in the mouth it is broken down mechanically and chemically. Chewing also activates the coordination of the sequential processes of the digestive tract that includes preparing an optimal insulin response and preparing to send signals of fullness back to the brain. Juicing provides large amounts of fructose and calories without the natural fibre. It has been suggested that our gut microbes are less well able to adapt to high doses of sugar in liquid form. There is also an adaptation to an overabundance of exotic fruits in a short time period and our fruits and vegetables are selectively bred for sweetness. High levels of fructose can overwhelm the digestive system and pass into the large intestine where it acts as a food source for the gut microbes. It is rapidly fermented into acids and gases, which cause common symptoms such as bloating, diarrhoea, constipation, tummy aches and flatulence.

Blended drinks with vegetables and some fat are preferable as the speed of sugar absorption is slower. Try to keep the consistency of blended drinks thick and to drink slowly. It is even better to consume soups that are 'eaten' in the mouth. This allows for increased digestion in the mouth.

Fruit

Avoid eating fruit at the end of a meal as it leads to fermentation in the gut. If you are snacking on fruit in the morning or drinking fresh juice, combine with a handful of nuts and seeds to slow down the absorption of carbohydrate to help control blood sugar. High-fructose fruit, such as dried fruit, grapes, pears, cherries, apples, watermelon and mangoes, can contribute to digestive problems such as bloating. The extent of this can vary according to your individual tolerance of individual foods.

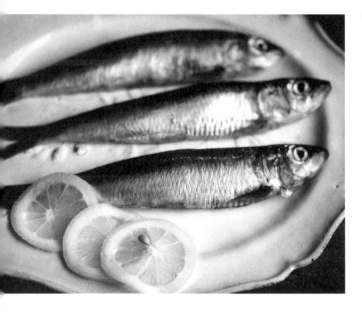

Fish and heavy metals

Heavy metals, such as lead, mercury and cadmium, are present in the environment, and enter the human body through contamination from food packaging, dental amalgams and consumption of larger fish such as tuna. Research suggests that high levels of heavy metals in blood can reduce fertility[1] and mercury found in contaminated fish sources may affect both sperm and fetal development.[2] However, omega-3 oil present in oily fish may play an important positive role in fertility by delaying ovarian ageing and improving egg quality.[3] According to one study[4] the health benefits of eating oily fish outweigh the danger of exposure to mercury. So my advice is to eat oily fish because it has many health benefits, but eat smaller fish such as mackerel and sardines and limit your servings of larger fish to once a week. If you do eat larger fish, removing the fat and skin may help to reduce traces of metals.

Soya and flaxseed

Phytoestrogens are plant-based hormones that have the potential for weak oestrogenic or anti-oestrogenic effects in the body that alter the natural hormone balance. There are many plants that contain phytoestrogens but the highest concentrations are found in soya and flaxseeds.

Some animal studies suggest that large amounts of soya in the diet may negatively affect fertility. It has been proposed that women with subfertility may be more sensitive to soya. There are also studies suggesting that the phytoestrogens from soya products lower sperm counts. We know that there are countries where soya is consumed and the birth rate is comparable to other countries but the way we consume soya here is very different. In the East, soya beans are typically consumed as whole foods. I advocate avoiding soya products when trying to conceive. Remember that people may believe their diets to be low in soya but it is added to many processed foods including chocolate, bread, protein shakes and bars and ready-made meals.

At the same dosage the oestrogenic effects in the body are greater from flaxseed than from soya. In 2008 a large Canadian study found that consumption of flaxseed oil (not seeds) was associated with an increased risk of miscarriage and premature birth. Avoid consuming flaxseed oil and check ingredient lists carefully. Flaxseeds (as part of a seed mix) can be eaten sparingly.

Artificial sweeteners, stabilisers, emulsifiers and preservatives

Artificial sweeteners, stabilisers, emulsifiers and preservatives are deemed safe for human consumption. However, research suggests that their effect on the diversity of gut microbes (reducing beneficial microbes) may have significance for human health and they are associated with potentially harmful metabolic effects including inflammation, obesity and metabolic syndrome. In some people these additives can cause gastrointestinal side effects that include bloating, gas, cramping and diarrhoea.

By their nature, artificial sweeteners encourage sugar craving and sugar dependence. Animal studies suggest that artificial sweeteners are associated with decreased red blood cells, male infertility (by lowering sperm count), enlarged kidneys and increase in miscarriage rates. Look out for artificial sweeteners in fizzy drinks and other soft drinks (including sports drinks), sweets, chewing gum, some medicines (for example, hayfever syrups and even some fertility supplements) and tonic waters.

Artificial sweeteners typically found in chewing gum are aspartame, sucralose (Splenda), sorbitol, saccharine and mannitol. If you are chewing gum to cure bad breath (rather than out of habit), one alternative for refreshing the breath is to use a drop of food-grade peppermint oil (real peppermint, not flavouring) on the tongue. There are some naturally sweetened chewing gums on the market but, with or without artificial sweeteners, chewing gum sends signals that activate enzymes and acids. When the anticipated food does not arrive there is an increased insulin release, increased gastric emptying and the release of digestive hormones.

Sugar

The creation of refined sugars and the addition of hidden sugars to our food is one of the biggest nutritional disasters of our time; its impact is only just being realised.

The dangers of excess sugar consumption were proposed by John Yudkin in the 1980s, when the rest of the world was continuing its love affair with low-fat diets. Scientific studies dating back from the late 1940s seemed to demonstrate that high-fat diets, and particularly high cholesterol, were causing heart disease. By the 1960s low fat was being adopted by everyone, not just by high-risk heart patients. By the 1980s low fat was in the mainstream consciousness, supported by government, medics, health media and the food industry.

At the same time in England in 1986 John Yudkin, author of *Pure, White and Deadly,* proposed that glucose alters our metabolic processes and increases plasma concentration of cholesterol and triglycerides. This leads to an increase in size of the liver, kidneys and adrenal glands. It causes calcified deposits on the kidneys. Furthermore, it disrupts oestrogen levels, adrenals, cortisol and insulin. Instead of listening to Yudkin's message about sugar, physicians and governments continued to go with the cholesterol and saturated fat hypothesis and soon the food industry was taking fat out of everything. In order to make the food palatable without the fat they laced the food with hidden sugars, and the rest is history. Well, actually the rest is: obesity, infertility, heart disease, diabetes and increased risks of cancer and autoimmune diseases.

Sweet-flavoured foods are actually the most nourishing of all foods. These include pumpkin, squash and carrots. They help the digestive system function and can provide great energy to the body. Some sweet flavour in the diet is essential. However, given the amount of sugar hidden in foods and the levels at which it is consumed, we nearly all greatly exceed our requirement for the sweet stuff.

In terms of fertility, you need to be careful of all forms of sugar as they all impact on blood sugar levels and on insulin. Research demonstrates that high blood sugars and insulin levels impact on egg quality. Women with high blood sugar and insulin levels consistently produce lower quality and fewer eggs during IVF, with lower implantation rates. High blood sugar and insulin also result in more miscarriages.[5] Sugar causes Dampness to form in the body – I will never forget one of my Chinese Medicine Masters telling us, 'Sugar will make the ovaries form cysts.'

Fruit contains fructose and glucose and although this has the same effect as other less healthy forms of sugar, it does at least have some benefits to health and fertility. When eating fruit limit your portions to one a day, eat early in the day and pick fruit with a low GI: berries, apples and pears are the best choices for balancing blood sugars (*see page 91*).

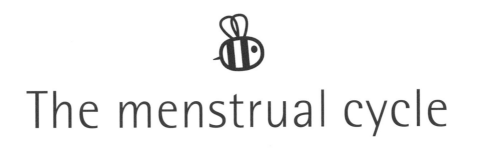

The menstrual cycle

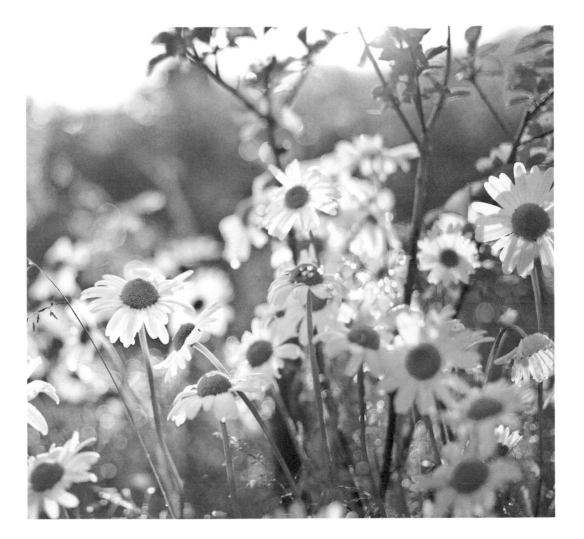

'The ebb and flow of dreams, creativity, and hormones associated with different parts of the cycle offer us a profound opportunity to deepen our connection with our inner knowing.'
Christiane Northrup, MD, *Women's Bodies, Women's Wisdom*

Our bodies are incredible and go through cycles every month of growth, development and renewal. Deep inside you a miraculous process happens time and again, in preparation for when you are ready to have a baby. Our amazing menstrual cycle is the aspect of us that makes us female and that gives us our fertility. Sadly, for many this is something that is not celebrated; either because you have never been encouraged to connect with it, or because it is a source of pain in your life.

I want to help you engage in and support your body in this miraculous process, whether you want to have a baby now or at some point in the future; you never know when you will decide the time is right. You never know when your body will be called upon to perform the amazing job of conceiving and carrying a baby. Your menstrual cycle is the only outward sign you have that your body is fertile. I think this is something very precious that needs to be valued and understood. Not just when we are ready, but throughout our lives. This is what I teach my children and this is what I want to teach you now.

Know and honour your body. This is the starting point for a fertile life and although it is a wonderful thing to have had a life-long relationship with your body it is never too late to start to treat it well and to make fertile choices every day.

Be your own guru

For a long time now we have relied heavily on others to direct us with our health; doctors, consultants, experts and gurus. There is nothing wrong with consulting an expert and going for regular checkups. But we have become overly reliant on external forces and do not invest enough time in what I call 'our internal landscape'. I encourage you to become your own guru and by that I mean develop your own intuition and inner knowing. Learn to trust your 'gut feelings'; they often come from a very wise place inside you – a place that knows what is best for you, better than I know or anyone else knows.

Learning about your body through the signs and feelings that you experience during the different phases of your menstrual cycle is an excellent place to start. It is said that a good practitioner can tell everything they need to know about a woman's health and fertility through observing her menstrual cycle. I spend most of my days observing and analysing my patients' fertility through the information I glean from menstrual symptoms. There is no reason why you cannot become a mini expert on your own body by analysing your own symptoms.

Remember, being your own guru does not mean becoming ultra-vigilant. It is much more about developing self-awareness.

Menstrual signs

	Sign	Tendency
Colour of menstrual blood	Dark red or bright red	Too much Heat (normally in the blood)
	Blackish	Blood Stagnation
	Pale	Blood Deficient
	Purple	Cold (and/or Cold uterus)
Pain	Stabbing pain like a knife	Blood Stagnation
	Pain that is better with the application of heat	Too much Cold
	Pain when the period ends	Blood Deficient
	Pre-menstrual pain	Stagnation
	Pain with heavy feeling	Damp
	Pain at ovulation	Heat and Damp combined
	Cramps	Too much Cold
	Pain dragging	Weak energy
Other features	Clotted blood	Blood Stagnation
	Clotted and dark blood	Too much Cold
	Watery or lack of blood	Blood Deficient
	Blood with mucus	Damp
	PMS	Stagnation of Qi
	Headaches	Too much Heat
	Bloating	Stagnation of Qi
	Tender breasts	Stagnation of Qi
Length of cycle	Anything from 28 to 32 days in length is deemed normal, although ideally the cycle is 28 days	
Regularity of cycle	Consistently early (a cycle of 23 days or less)	Heat
	Consistently late (a cycle of 33 days or more)	Blood Stagnation, and/or too much Cold
	Irregular	Stagnation of Qi

Menstrual Optimisation Plan

I have devised the Menstrual Optimisation Plan to help women engage with and optimise their menstrual cycle and their fertility. It is best suited to women who have a regular cycle. If your cycle is irregular, I suggest that you start with the Menstrual Tonic (*see page 52*), which may help to regulate it. If your cycle is persistently irregular you can subtly adapt the phases of the Optimisation Plan to work for you.

- I encourage my patients to start to keep a simple diary or journal where they record the days of their cycle.
- Start to engage in your cycle and observe the ebb and flow.
- Day one of your cycle is the day the period starts. Mark this in your diary as 'Day 1'. If the period starts in the afternoon or evening, then the following day is 'Day 1'.
- Make a note of the length of the cycle.
- Make notes about how you feel at each phase.
- Observe your physical symptoms, for example, what day do you notice secretions, do you have pain, and so on.
- Consider what is the nature of the period itself (*see Menstrual Signs box, page 45*).

'MOVE' phase: Days 1–5/7 (approx.)

Making sure the Blood and the Qi moves well at this phase is the focus at this time. This is when lots of oestrogen is being produced and when follicles in the ovary begin to grow to be released at ovulation. The endometrium is shedding. Although conventional physicians do not place much importance on the flow and quality of the period, diagnostically it offers a unique insight into the health and fertility of the woman (*see Menstrual Signs box, page 45*).

It is important that the endometrium is fully shed and so foods that encourage the regulation and movement of Blood and Qi are eaten at this stage. Gentle exercise is also helpful as movement will support the expulsion of the uterus lining. But do not excessively exercise during your period or get cold.

Many patients will notice a change in their menstrual bleed after making adjustments. Typically, the blood will flow more easily, be more red and less clotted.

BLOOD-MOVING FOODS

Aubergines, chestnuts, chilli, chives, crab, eggs, kohlrabi, leeks, liver, mustard leaf, onions, peaches, radishes, saffron, spring onions, sticky rice, turmeric and vinegar.

Phases of the menstrual cycle

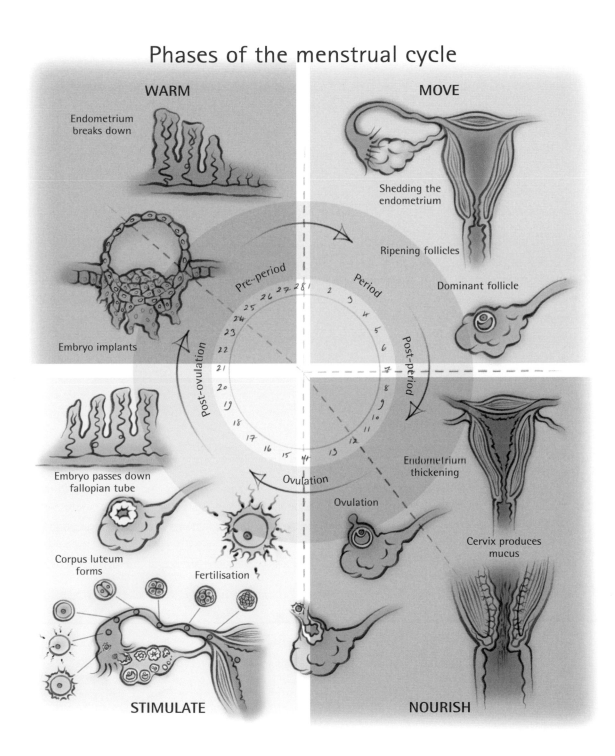

BLOOD-NOURISHING FOODS

Aduki beans, apricots, beef, beetroot, bone marrow, cherries, dandelion, dates, eggs, figs, grapes, kale, kidney beans, leafy greens, mussels, nettle, octopus, oysters, parsley, sardines, seaweed, squid, sweet rice, tempeh and watercress.

YIN-NOURISHING FOODS

Apples, asparagus, avocados, cheese, clams, crab, duck, eggs, green beans, honey, lemons, malt, mangoes, milk, nettles, oysters, pears, pineapple, pomegranates, pork, seaweed, sesame seeds, spelt, spinach, tomatoes, watermelon, wheat and yam.

'NOURISH' phase: Days 7–13 (approx.)

As soon as the bleeding has stopped (this will be slightly different in everyone, but between days 5-7) it is time to nourish the body by eating Blood- and Yin-nourishing foods. The dominant follicle is maturing in the ovary and will be released at ovulation. The lining of the womb is also thickening, and the cervix is beginning to produce fertile mucus.

Rest and nourishing foods are key now. Foods that support Blood and Yin can help support follicle development and ultimately the quality of the egg that is produced. Of course we are not talking about changing DNA here, but the energetic integrity of the egg can be influenced.

'STIMULATE' phase: Days 14–18/19 (approx.)

In this phase of the cycle the focus is firstly on the release of a mature egg at ovulation and secondly on its smooth passage down the fallopian tubes. Much of fertility is about good transportation and this requires good movement.

The emotions are also important at this phase; being relaxed and not rigidly focusing on pinpointing ovulation is key. Rigidity can cause a great deal of stagnation in the body and prevent an egg from being released. If there is too much stagnation then the uterus also becomes tense and

STIMULATING FOODS

Almonds, caraway, cardamom, carrots, cayenne, chicken, coconut, dates, eggs, fennel seeds, figs, grapes, lentils, millet, molasses, oats, quinoa, rice, sage, sardines, shiitake mushrooms, star anise, squash and tangerine peel.

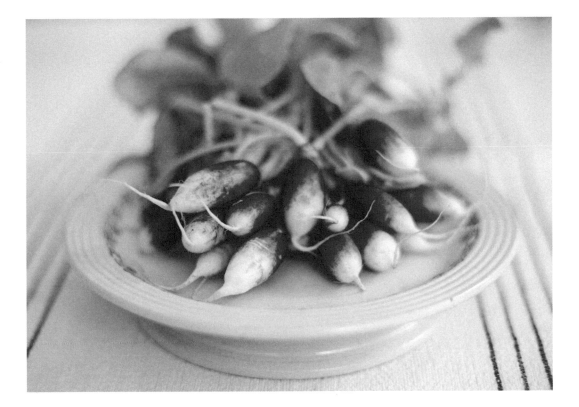

not open enough to receive the sperm. So having a relaxed attitude and being ready to receive the sperm, and ultimately an embryo, will help at this stage.

Eat well in the morning; oats are ideal. In the evening, eat lightly – remember you will need to keep your libido strong at this stage of the month and eating a heavy meal will make you tired. Also, going to bed after too much food will make the system very stagnant, which is the opposite of what we are trying to achieve here.

Do not become fixated on foods and timings of sex as this will cause Stagnation in the system. Instead be more spontaneous and enjoy yourself. Sex to order is no fun and it will achieve the opposite of what you are aiming for.

'WARM' phase: Days 20–28 (approx.)

The importance of a warm womb has been advocated by physicians of Chinese medicine for thousands of years. Old texts of Chinese medicine describe how a cold uterus can cause infertility; a warm uterus supports implantation. Certainly in clinic I encourage women to keep warm during this phase of the

> ## WARMING FOODS
>
> Almonds, beetroot, carrots, cayenne pepper, chicken, chocolate, cinnamon, cloves, figs, garlic, ginger, lamb, mustard, nutmeg, peaches, peppers, pumpkin, radishes, sesame seeds, squash and tomatoes (cooked).

cycle. If the abdomen is cold to touch I encourage practices that warm the body. This includes eating warming foods, keeping the feet and midriff warm, avoiding draughts and avoiding cold foods and drink.

Implantation: 8–10 days after ovulation

If the egg has been fertilised by sperm and has become an embryo, it will implant in the lining of the uterus. If the embryo arrives too late it may fail to implant. Embryos that implant at Day 11 post ovulation as more likely to fail.

No implantation

If no implantation takes place the endometrium will break down and be shed as the period.

Menstrual disorders

Many problems I see in women in their thirties can be traced back to their twenties. A problem that starts at that age may develop into a bigger problem later in life when it may be harder to treat and may impact on fertility. It is very important for younger women to develop an awareness of their bodies and cycles in their twenties so that they can preserve their fertility.

No periods is one of the most common issues and can come about from weight loss, over-exercise, adrenal stress, burn out, emotional stress or because of polycystic ovary syndrome (PCOS). It may seem great in your twenties not to have a period but it is a sign that your body is not functioning properly and that your hormones are out of balance. Our bodies are well designed and give us warning signs; learning to observe your menstrual symptoms is a great way to learn about your body.

Polycystic ovary syndrome

This is a condition characterised by multiple small cysts on the ovaries, which normally results in longer cycles due to delayed ovulation. It may also result in acne and facial hair. This condition may be full blown or it may be mild where the ovaries have a cystic appearance but regular ovulation still takes place. Having PCOS does not necessarily make you infertile, particularly if you are still ovulating. However, if you have very long cycles you are probably not ovulating regularly, which will reduce your chances of conception. If you are overweight and you have PCOS, losing weight may help. (This is a fascinating observation as in the general population – in other words, those without PCOS genes – losing weight is normally associated with periods and ovulation stopping.)

Diagnosis
PCOS always involves an element of Dampness and Stagnation (*see pages 31–32 and 35–36*). My main aim in treatment is to try to establish ovulation by moving Stagnation and eliminating Damp-forming foods. Regular exercise is recommended. Acupuncture is also a very reliable treatment to stimulate ovulation. Follow the Optimisation Plan and do a full month. For those that do not bleed, the day of the next full moon can be taken as Day 1.

Endometriosis
In endometriosis endometrial tissue is found outside of the uterus, in the pelvic cavity (and sometimes in other areas of the body). It is thought to impact on fertility in several ways:
- It may block the fallopian tubes or impact on the function of the ovaries.
- Macrophages activity caused by the endometriosis may kill off sperm and prevent it from reaching the egg. This can be an issue if the sperm count is low.
- There may be a problem with the release of an egg and the transport of the egg via the fallopian tube at ovulation due to changes in the fertile mucus and prostaglandins, which support the function of the fallopian tubes.

Diagnosis
Follow the Blood Stagnation eating suggestions (*see page 37*) as well as doing the Body-Mind-Gut Programme (*see pages 72–80*). Follow this with the Menstrual Tonic (*see page 52*).

Stagnation of Qi and endometriosis caused by suppressed emotions and frustration may cause widespread Stagnation of energy resulting in abdominal cramps. Women affected often do not expel the endometrium sufficiently during their period and the blood is likely to travel upwards into the tubes. In some cases, particularly when the system is Cold and sluggish then the tissue stagnates and progresses to Blood Stagnation, which is present in endometriosis. So, as well as addressing the diet, it is also necessary to work on an emotional level to work on the reasons behind the frustration and suppressed emotions and to try to bring some of the hidden issues to the surface to be resolved.

Amenorrhoea
Amenorrhoea is the absence of periods, whether they never started at all (primary amenorrhoea) or they stopped at some point. If you do not have periods for several months you should visit your physician for further investigations.

Diagnosis

The causes of amenorrhoea are many and varied and beyond the scope of this book. However, it is worth doing the Menstrual Tonic, or full Optimisation Plan, even if you are not having a bleed. Sometimes what I do with my patients is choose the next full moon to be Day 1 and then follow the Menstrual Tonic eating plan from there. Do it for 28 days and then start again. Additionally, acupuncture has been shown to stimulate ovulation and would be a useful addition.

There is often a deficiency of Yin and Blood, which means the follicles do not reach maturity during the follicular phase of the cycle. By following the Menstrual Tonic you will help build Blood and Yin. Additionally, Damp and Blood Stagnation can prevent an egg from being released at mid cycle, which is why acupuncture works really well.

Exercise that encourages good movement in the hip and midriff, such as hula hooping or dancing, would also be helpful. If you identified with Damp or Blood Stagnation tendencies (*see pages 31 and 37*) look at the dietary suggestions and incorporate them in the Stimulate and Move phase of the cycle.

Fibroids

This is a condition of Blood Stagnation and, depending on the size and position of the fibroids, they may need to be surgically removed. However, following the dietary recommendations for Blood Stagnation is well worth doing regardless of whether you need to have them surgically removed or not. Often the Blood Stagnation has come about on a background of Coldness in the uterus so look at this as well and follow the suggestions for removing Cold.

Dysmenorrhoea

This condition, painful periods, will respond well to the Menstrual Tonic. The emphasis is on nourishing Blood in the follicular phase and moving Stagnant Qi and Blood in the luteal phase.

Menorrhagia

Heavy periods will also respond well to the Menstrual Tonic. Note if they include too much Heat. If this is the case the menstrual blood with be bright red.

The Menstrual Tonic

This seven-day cure is based on healing traditions from the East. In Asian countries many women recognise the importance of eating certain foods, particularly post period, in order to bring balance back to the menstrual cycle. The menstrual cycle is viewed as an important aspect of a woman's health, and food is a valuable tool to help bring the body back into balance.

I have witnessed many, many times how this simple tonic can transform a woman's entire menstrual cycle. In periods that have been stop/start the menstrual blood comes in with a good flow.

Periods can become normal with reduced pre-menstrual syndrome, or the blood becomes clearer – brighter, less clotted. I sometimes use this tonic between IVF cycles and see improvement in the quality of the womb lining or in the follicle growth in the following IVF cycle.

Throughout the Menstrual Tonic, add more of the following to recipes wherever you can:

- Chicken Broth Flavoured with Darkened Ginger (*see page 142*). Drink this on each day of the menu plan. It warms and nourishes the blood of the uterus.
- Black sesame oil (or regular sesame oil if black is difficult to find); this nourishes Blood and Yin.
- Rice wine to warm and move (for all but those who are too Hot).
- Eggs to nourish Blood and Yin.

For each stage of the Menstrual Optimisation Plan, include into your diet as many of the foods that are listed below as you can, or follow the menu plan (*see pages 56–57*).

Stage One: Days 1–2 of period
Invigorate, move and then nourish the Blood.

- Eat liver once each day – or steak if you cannot eat liver.
- **Other Blood-moving foods include**: aubergines, chestnuts, chilli, chives, crab, eggs, kohlrabi, leeks, mustard leaf, onions, peaches, radishes, saffron, spring onions, sticky rice, turmeric and vinegar.
- The most important adjustment to make during Days 1–2 is to increase rest by reducing exercise and getting one hour extra of sleep per night. It is also important to keep warm, so no walking on floorboards or stone floors in bare feet.

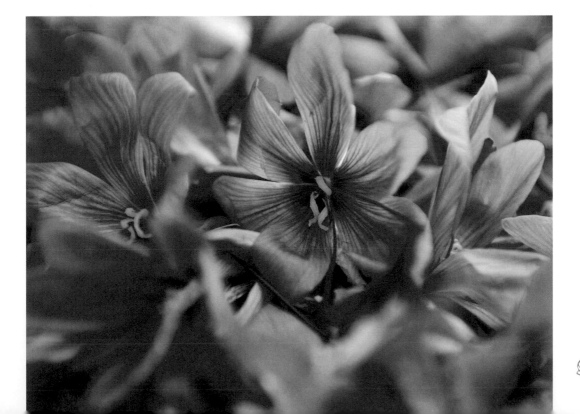

Stage Two: Days 3–4
Strengthen the Kidney energy.
- Eat kidneys once a day.
- **Other kidney-nourishing foods include**: alfalfa, asparagus, chestnuts, eggs, kidney beans, nettles, oats, quinoa, string beans and walnuts. Raspberry leaf tea is also helpful.
- **Essential oil**: using rose oil diluted in almond oil to rub onto the abdomen is a great tonic for the female reproductive system at this time.

Stage Three: Days 5–7
Tonify the whole body, especially the Qi, Blood and Yin.
- Eat chicken, ideally the Dang Gui Chicken Soup (*see page 143*).
- **Other Qi-nourishing foods include**: almonds, aromatic seeds (caraway, cardamom, coriander fennel), carrots, cherries, chickpeas, coconut, eggs, lentils, liquorice, mackerel, milk, millet, molasses, oats, potatoes, quinoa, rice, sage, sardines, sweet potatoes, shiitake mushrooms, squash, tofu, trout, venison and yam.
- **Other Blood-nourishing foods include**: aduki beans, apricots, beef, beetroot, bone marrow, cherries, dandelion, dates, eggs, figs, grapes, kale, kidney beans, leafy greens, mussels, nettle, octopus, oysters, parsley, sardines, seaweed, squid, sweet rice, tempeh and watercress.
- **Other Yin-nourishing foods include**: apple, asparagus, avocado, cheese, clams, crab, duck, eggs, green beans, honey, lemon, malt, mango, milk, nettle, oyster, pear, pineapple, pomegranate, pork, seaweed, sesame, spelt, spinach, tomato, watermelon, wheat and yam.

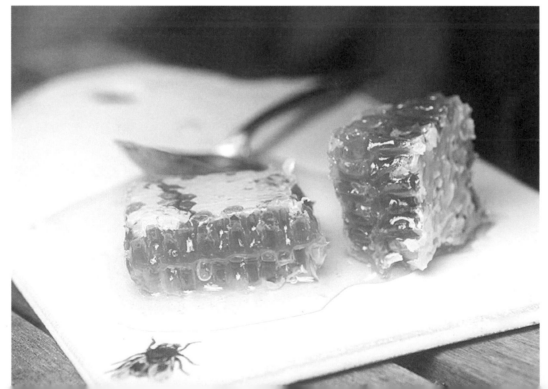

Sex and libido

When our reproductive system is functioning optimally and the cycle is regular then the libido too will be healthy. Everyone has a different quality to their libido and it is also dependent on the relationship dynamic. Most women when in good health will find they are more aroused around the time they are ovulating. Nature is a clever mistress and we are designed to want more sex when we are most fertile – we are also more attractive to the opposite sex at this time.

- In a 28-day cycle making love every 1–3 days throughout the cycle is optimal.
- Avoid using lubricants, oil or saliva as this can damage sperm or impact on the motility of sperm and its ability to travel through the cervix.
- Some traditions advocate preserving sperm by waiting until ovulation to enhance the potency of the sperm. This is not advised in modern practice as sperm benefits from frequent ejaculation. The only exception would be when the sperm count is low.[1]
- Oxytocin released during orgasm, which strengthens tubal contractions, helps sperm move through the fallopian tubes.
- Although charting the menstrual cycle can be helpful in order to identify the time of ovulation, over-focusing on such timing can cause anxiety in both partners.
- Couples who routinely use ovulation predictor kits have less sex and more sexual performance-related anxiety than couples that do not use them.
- Research has shown that stress impacts libido and is a factor in couples taking a prolonged time to conceive.
- Poor gut health impacts serotonin synthesis, which affects sexual desire and function (*see Fertile in Mind-Body-Gut, pages 69–84*).
- Semen contains large amounts of zinc so if you are having lots of sex it is a good idea to keep high levels of this in the body. Seeds tend to be high in zinc, particularly pumpkin and sesame seeds.

Food and libido

A lot has been made about libido-enhancing qualities of foods and certain nutrients; I think this is an area that needs some caution. It isn't as if you can eat a plate of oysters and then turn into Casanova. That said, I think eating food together can be a very pleasurable and sensual experience. Making a commitment to spend time in the pleasure of eating is far more important than stressing over cooking an ultra fertility-boosting, libido-enhancing meal. There is little more attractive than another person knowing your likes and taking pleasure in providing you with the things that make you happy. Spend time on setting the scene, making the room look pretty, lighting a few candles. Attention to detail and care in preparing the meal and the mood are more likely to improve libido than the content of the food. Light food is the best choice as a heavy meal can cause Stagnation and a reduction in libido.

Menstrual Optimisation menu plan

DAY	BREAKFAST	LUNCH	DINNER	SUGGESTED SNACKS
1	Warm water with lemon *and* scrambled eggs with Nut, Spice & Seed Mix (*see page 168*)	Fragrant Aubergines (*see page 188*)	Moroccan- spiced Chicken Livers (*see page 172*) with seasonal greens **Vegetarian option:** Butternut Squash, Chestnut & Seaweed Risotto (*see page 196*)	Chicken Broth Flavoured with Darkened Ginger (*see page 142*) Beetroot Soup (*see page 144*) Kefir Yoghurt Pot (*see page 211*) Turmeric Milk (*see page 212*)
2	Warm water with lemon *and* Black Sesame Porridge with Roasted Saffron Peaches (*see page 136*) served with a handful of pumpkin seeds	Baked Eggs with Vegetables (*see page 140*)	Pork & Chicken Liver Meatballs (*see page 173*) served with wilted greens **Vegetarian option:** Caponata with Toasted Almonds (*see page 189*)	Chicken Broth Flavoured with Darkened Ginger (*see page 142*) Beetroot Soup (*see page 144*) Kefir Yoghurt Pot (*see page 211*) Turmeric Milk (*see page 212*)
3	Warm water with lemon *and* scrambled eggs with steamed asparagus	Three-bean Tagine with Almond & Lemon Couscous (*see page 192*)	Stir-fried Kidneys with Ginger & Sesame (*see page 174*) **Vegetarian option:** Roasted vegetables with Walnut Tarator Sauce (*see page 165*)	Chicken Broth Flavoured with Darkened Ginger (*see page 142*) Beetroot Soup (*see page 144*) Kefir Yoghurt Pot (*see page 211*) Turmeric Milk (*see page 212*)
4	Warm water with lemon *and* Sweet Chestnut Congee (*see page 207*)	Kidney Bean, Quinoa & Leek Salad with Toasted Pumpkin Seeds (*see page 195*)	Kidneys & Mushrooms in a Creamy Mustard Sauce with Puy Lentils (*see page 175*) **Vegetarian option:** Sweet Potato & Chickpea Gnocchi (*see page 200*) with Walnut & Rocket Pesto (*see page 166*)	Chicken Broth Flavoured with Darkened Ginger (*see page 142*) Beetroot Soup (*see page 144*) Kefir Yoghurt Pot (*see page 211*) Turmeric Milk (*see page 212*)

DAY	BREAKFAST	LUNCH	DINNER	SUGGESTED SNACKS
5	Warm water with lemon *and* 'Carrot Cake' Overnight Oats (*see page 138*)	Oyster, Leek & Sweet Potato Soup with Japanese 7-spice Powder (*see page 146*) **Vegetarian option**: Dahl with Roasted Tomatoes (*see page 154*)	Beetroot & Coconut Curry (*see page 194*)	Dang Gui Chicken Soup (see page 143) Beetroot Soup (*see page 144*) Kefir Yoghurt Pot (*see page 211*) Turmeric Milk (*see page 212*)
6	Warm water with lemon *and* scrambled eggs with sliced avocado	Baked Feta with Vegetable Spaghetti (*see page 202*)	Beef Shin & Pumpkin Stew (*see page 181*) **Vegetarian option**: Three-bean Tagine with Almond & Lemon Couscous (*see page 192*)	Dang Gui Chicken Soup (*see page 143*) Beetroot Soup (*see page 144*) Kefir Yoghurt Pot (*see page 211*) Turmeric Milk (*see page 212*)
7	Warm water with lemon *and* Quinoa, Chia Seed & Cardamom Porridge with Coconut, Pistachios & Raspberries *(see page 134)*	Chicken, Asparagus & Tarragon Soup (*see page 151*) **Vegetarian option**. Aduki Bean, Tomato & Miso Soup (*see page 148*)	Roasted Sardines with Tomato, Onion & Pomegranate (*see page 177*) **Vegetarian option**: Spiced Paneer with Wilted Greens (*see page 199*)	Dang Gui Chicken Soup (*see page 143*) Beetroot Soup (*see page 144*) Kefir Yoghurt Pot (*see page 211*) Turmeric Milk (*see page 212*)

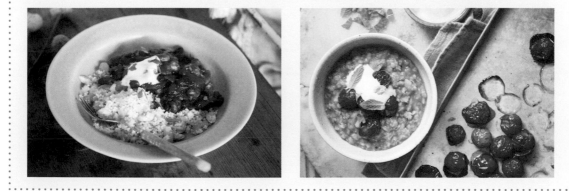

Do

- Spend time making an effort, choose favourite foods and include some element of adventurousness.
- Relax and enjoy the experience and be in the moment – being present and attentive is very attractive.
- Remember that food is a sensual experience enhanced by sharing.

Don't

- Drink too much or eat too much or stress about the meal.
- Spend too much time on complicated dishes that keep you in the kitchen instead of with your partner.
- Obsess about what you are eating; it's not attractive to be too self-absorbed.

Holistic approach

Libido is a complex aspect of a person and an area that, when probed, is likely to bring up some difficult emotions. Sometimes there is a lack of libido due to tiredness, gut health or nutritional issues, but it may be that it has its root in emotional causes. Trying for a baby can bring pressure into the relationship, particularly if it does not happen easily. There can be self-blame or -loathing, feelings of shame and inadequacy, or just the sheer pressure of having to perform. It is important to try and prevent issues from arising. Remember that trying for a baby is a loving expression of your union. Spend time relaxing together and if libido is an issue try massaging one another. If it continues to be an issue seek help from your GP. Don't turn baby making into a chore and don't schedule sex into 'fertile days'; this quickly builds the pressure and creates performance-related anxiety.

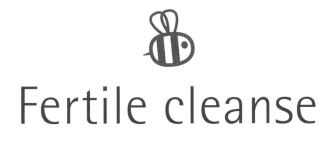

Fertile cleanse

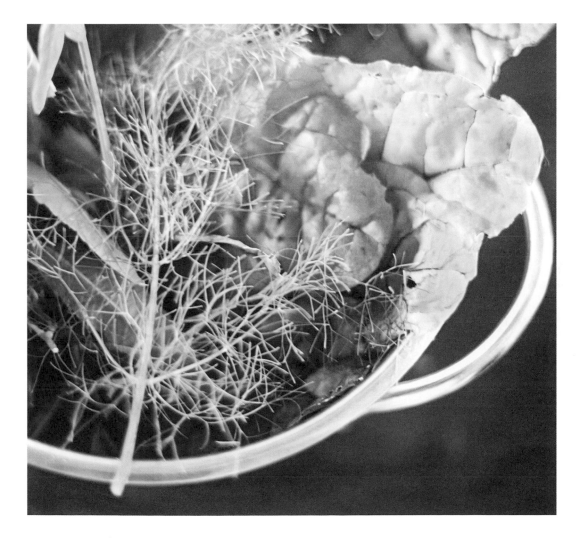

I want you to see the Fertile Cleanse as a diet cleanse rather than as a detox. It is a way of introducing you to a more healthy and fertile style of eating. It can help you to break harmful habits as well as introduce new and delicious ways of eating into your diet.

Simplifying the diet, purging or simply abstaining from certain foods is part of many traditional healing traditions. In the 1930s Dr Mayr, an Austrian physician, discovered while treating men on the battlefields that they got better much more quickly if they abstained from food or simplified their diet for a period of time in order to encourage the healing process.

The purpose of a diet cleanse is in part to rest the digestion and so for that reason I advocate three meals a day with a long gap between dinner and breakfast. Don't forget breakfast gets its name from 'breaking the fast'. Dinner needs to be eaten as early as possible so that the body has fasted for a long period of time through the night. This means eating a light dinner by 7pm.

Sometimes when we need to start to introduce new eating habits a bit of preparation helps us to focus. This isn't about guilt and sacrifice and it isn't about being perfect!

The Fertile Cleanse takes one week and is of benefit in the following circumstances:

• You want to break some bad habits like smoking or excessive drinking.
• You are doing the Body-Mind-Gut Programme (*see pages 72–80*).
• You are trying to cut sugar and other anti-nutrients out of your diet.
• As preparation for IVF or following a failed IVF.
• As a seasonal adjustment; Spring or Autumn is the best time.

Introducing fertile habits – getting started

Deciding to start trying for a baby can be exciting and nerve-racking in equal measure. It is important not to get into the mind-set of: 'OK, darling, we are trying NOW!' It immediately puts pressure on the situation. Increasingly though, this is the mind-set of many modern couples who are used to planning and scheduling every last detail of their hectic lives. A gentle word of advice is not to PLAN to make a baby; instead I want you to think about it in terms of preparation. Things may happen easily, or they may take a little longer, and the more wedded to your plan you are the harder it will be to be flexible and resourceful if things don't go to schedule! You see that is the problem with a plan – great if it works, very bad if it doesn't.

It is rather like the Buddhist idea of holding on 'not too tight, not too loose'. When we hold a musical instrument too tightly the strings break, yet if we hold too loosely, no sound comes out. It is the same with fertility; you need to engage in it, yet keep a lightness to your touch – if you focus on it too greatly you will create tensions, but if you hold it too loosely you will let it slip through your fingers. So the trick is to engage, yet remain soft and yielding.

This is a good attitude to take when buying food. I find the best way to approach food shopping is to have a few ideas of what you would like to cook and then see what is on offer. That way you can be flexible and adapt to what you are presented with, following the path of your heart a little when you see something fertile- and fresh-looking that may not have been what you wrote on your list.

I suggest you approach your baby making in much the same way. Decide gently on an emotional level that you and your partner are happy to start thinking and preparing for a baby. When you make this decision I suggest you don't immediately start working out when this baby will be born and if that month is convenient for you. I also recommend you don't work out what star sign you want for a child or if that is a good month to be born in order to do well at school! Believe me, I have seen all of the above scenarios.

I also suggest you don't immediately overhaul your entire life by stripping away all the fun things you do as a couple and removing all the foods you love to eat. This isn't about creating a joyless life for yourselves, it is about preparing for a baby, which is a thing of great joy and celebration. If you have been living a wild and carefree existence you will have to rein it in a little, but babies are not created through joyless control and denial.

So with that in mind I want you to set aside a month where you gently shift your focus to preparing for a baby. Imagine you are preparing a palace for the arrival of someone very special. You will want the place to be in tip-top condition and for everything to be functioning optimally.

Preparation

Go through your cupboards, larder, pantry or fridge and give them a bit of a sort out, getting rid of anything you would like to eliminate from your diet. I advise you to get rid of anything processed or packaged. Processed foods are often high in added sugars, contain cheap plant oils and contain food additives that have a detrimental effect on your microbes. These ingredients all contribute to intestinal inflammation with subsequent metabolic dysfunction. Next, stock up on tasty, healthy foods:

- Unprocessed wholegrains.
- Gluten-free grains: quinoa, buckwheat, oats, amaranth, teff.
- Grains containing gluten (if tolerated): spelt, barley, rye, freekeh.
- Legumes, chickpeas, lentils.
- Seeds: black and white sesame seeds, pumpkin, chia seeds, flaxseeds, sunflower.
- Nuts: almond, brazil nuts, walnuts.
- Tinned fish: sardines and anchovies.
- Herbal teas.
- Nut butters.
- Dried seaweed.
- Dried fruits: apricots, dates (unsulphured).
- Raw cacao.
- Oils: olive oil, coconut oil, hempseed oil, pumpkin oil, avocado oil.

Chicken broth and other bone broths

I am not happy unless I have chicken broth in the fridge and some frozen in ice-cube trays in the fridge. The best way to do this is to regularly boil chicken bones and make fresh stock to use and freeze (*see page 142*). The ice-cubes can be added frozen to dishes such as vegetables or stews to improve their nutritional value. A slightly easier way is to buy a good quality ready-made version, organic if possible (go for the liquid versions). This makes a perfect base for many dishes in this book.

A word about raw

As a practitioner of Chinese medicine, I have never been a massive fan of raw food. I see many patients who consume large amounts of raw food when they have a very compromised digestion. This is a common mistake as a weak digestion cannot digest raw food easily. However, there is nothing like a lovely salad in Summer or a fresh piece of fruit in the morning and so over the years I have adapted my take on raw food.

In the morning when the digestion is strong and the stomach energy is at its strongest, fruit and raw veg (as in smoothies) are well tolerated by most people. For those with a good digestion, so with no bloating, pain or flatulence, salad at lunch is fine. But very few people can digest raw food at night. What happens is that the raw food ferments in the intestines, producing alcohol, and this changes the lining of the gut and causes inflammation.

From a Chinese medicine understanding, it is said that an over-consumption of raw food actually causes digestive weakness and leads to Dampness in the body. I think it also needs to be borne in mind what the climate is like where you live – for example, in a cold, damp country the body will thrive on warm, cooked foods.

This is important when thinking about doing a cleanse, as people often think this means living off smoothies and juices. This is a mistake; there is nothing wrong with the odd juice, they taste great and on paper seem like a good option nutritionally. But as I explained on page 39, the problem with juices is they are actually 'overly nutritious' and they bypass the normal process of digestion – chewing! Chewing is a very important part of the digestive process; when we chew we improve the function of the liver and pancreas. We produce saliva and we help establish new neural pathways in the brain. When we drink juice, the juice arrives directly into the stomach unannounced. The stomach then has to work extra hard to digest this overly nutritious substance, putting an additional strain on the digestive process.

From my yearly studies with Dr Stossier of the world-famous Viva Mayr clinic in Austria, I have observed how women who suffer from fermentation also have distortion in the lower abdomen. The lower abdomen houses the intestines but also the reproductive organs: uterus, fallopian tubes and ovaries. When the fermentation is chronic there is inflammation and Stagnation in the reproductive

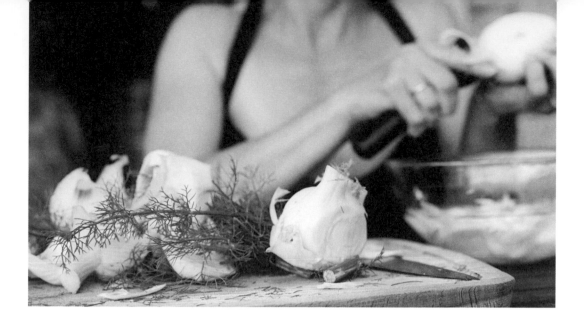

organs. The posture of the person changes in order to compensate for the distortion; they develop the 'duck posture' where the lower back becomes concave and the bottom sticks out. This may affect both movement and implantation. Patients who have this issue benefit from doing the Cleanse followed by the Body-Mind-Gut Programme (*see pages 72–80*).

The Cleanse

Once you are ready to start the Cleanse, follow the menu plan on pages 64–65. Begin each day with a drink of hot water with lemon juice added. Breakfast should be eggs, avocado or some ewe or goats' cheese on toasted rye bread, or alternatively porridge with seeds and butter (and a small amount of honey).

Lunch is the main meal of the day and should be bigger than dinner. It is fine to have raw food at lunch and some meat but make the protein portion of the meal the size of the palm of your hand (i.e. excluding the fingers). Do make sure you chew all foods very well, but particularly raw food. Think of your mouth as the first place of digestion and remember, the stomach does not have teeth! Sardines, chicken, turkey, steamed veg, oven-roasted veg, quinoa salad, amaranth, stir-fried leafy greens are examples of a good lunch.

Dinner must be eaten by 7pm. This is very important and having dinner early will ensure that your body is repairing overnight and not digesting. Don't forget: no raw food with dinner. Soup is ideal but it is also fine to have some vegetables or something else light. Try not to mix carbohydrates and protein as your body will find just one food type so much easier to digest.

Aim to drink two litres of water per day but not with meals. The water needs to be room temperature and not cold or with ice in it. Also drink as much herbal tea as you like throughout the day; this counts towards your hydration quota. Don't drink fruit juice. Coconut water is great when it's hot – make sure you buy unpasteurised, unflavoured coconut water. Filtered water is preferable to water bought and stored in plastic bottles, which are both environmentally unfriendly and potentially hormone disruptors due to the BPAs in the plastic.

Fertile Cleanse menu plan

DAY	BREAKFAST	LUNCH	DINNER	SUGGESTED SNACKS
1	Warm water with lemon *and* Simple Overnight Oats *(see page 138)* with mixed seeds, seasonal berries and a little raw honey to taste	Kidney Bean, Quinoa & Leek Salad with Toasted Pumpkin Seeds *(see page 195)* served with a little Naturally Fermented Sauerkraut *(see page 160)*	Carrot, Sweet Potato & Coriander Soup *(see page 149)*	Kefir Yoghurt Pot *(see page 211)* Chicken Broth *(see page 142)*
2	Warm water with lemon *and* scrambled eggs with sliced avocado	Saffron Fish & Vegetable Stew *(see page 180)* **Vegetarian option:** Spiced Paneer with Wilted Greens *(see page 199)*	Aduki Bean, Tomato and Miso soup *(see page 148)*	Cannonball (any) *(see pages 209–210)* Chicken Broth *(see page 142)*
3	Warm water with lemon *and* Simple Overnight Oats *(see page 138)* with blackberries, chopped hazelnuts and a little raw honey to taste	Almond-crusted Salmon with Cauliflower Purée *(see page 184)* served with wilted greens **Vegetarian option:** Baked Feta with Vegetable Spaghetti *(see page 202)*	Leek & Fennel Soup with Toasted Walnuts *(see page 152)*	Cannonball (any) *(see pages 209–210)* Chicken Broth *(see page 142)*
4	Warm water with lemon *and* Mixed Grain Porridge with Blackberries, Hazelnuts & Flaxseeds *(see page 133)*	Buckwheat Salad with Butternut Squash, Asparagus & Pecans *(see page 190)* served with raw fermented vegetables, such as Naturally Fermented Sauerkraut *(see page 160)*	Chicken, Asparagus & Tarragon Soup *(see page 151)* **Vegetarian option:** Lentil & Leafy Greens Soup *(see page 157)*	Kefir Yoghurt Pot *(see page 211)* Chicken Broth *(see page 142)*

DAY	BREAKFAST	LUNCH	DINNER	SUGGESTED SNACKS
5	Warm water with lemon *and* 'Carrot Cake' Overnight Oats (*see page 138*)	Beef, Broccoli & Quinoa Stir Fry (*see page 178*) **Vegetarian option:** Broccoli & Quinoa Stir Fry with Avocado & Toasted Cashews (*see page 198*)	Beetroot Soup (*see page 144*)	Cannonball (any) (*see pages 209–210*) Chicken Broth (*see page 142*)
6	Warm water with lemon *and* a poached egg with sautéed greens	Caponata with Toasted Almonds (*see page 189*)	Chicken Soup with Courgette Noodles (*see page 153*) **Vegetarian option:** Sweet Potato, Cavolo Nero & Almond Soup (*see page 156*)	Kefir Yoghurt Pot (*see page 211*) Chicken Broth (*see page 142*)
7	Warm water with lemon *and* Baked Porridge with Goji Berries & Cinnamon (*see page 135*)	Grilled Mackerel with Probiotic Kohlrabi & Fennel Coleslaw (*see page 176*) **Vegetarian option:** Dahl with Roasted Tomatoes (*see page 154*)	Celeriac & Chestnut Soup with Chestnut & Herb Pesto (*see page 147*)	Cannonball (any) (*see pages 209–210*) Chicken Broth (*see page 142*)

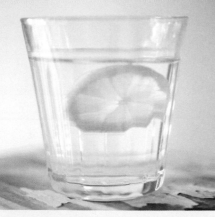

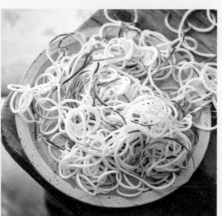

Rituals during the Cleanse

The Fertile Cleanse is not just about what you eat. Following some simple rituals during the week of the Cleanse will benefit your overall health. If you find some of these rituals particularly beneficial, you may wish to make them a part of your everyday routines.

Oil pulling

This is a cleansing technique originating from Ayurvedic medicine. It is simple yet incredibly powerful. So often when people decide to go on a health kick they attend to everything but their dental and oral hygiene. This is so important as infection in the mouth and gums can really impact on general health and can cause more systemic imbalances within the body.

Do this daily during the Cleanse, and three times per week thereafter. You will need cold-pressed olive oil, sesame oil or coconut oil. Allow an extra 10-20 minutes in your morning routine.

Swill one teaspoon of oil (I used organic coconut oil) around your mouth for 20 minutes once a day in the morning on an empty stomach. It's important to keep the oil moving around your mouth and to change the angle of your head every now and then in order that the oil reaches all the nooks and crannies. The liquid will increase in volume as it mixes with saliva and so it is important not to swallow any of it as it is drawing toxins out of the body. After 20 minutes spit the liquid out and rinse your mouth with some warm water and salt.

Dry skin brushing

Starting on the soles of the feet, use a body brush (a rounded wooden brush with soft bristles) to brush the skin. Always brush towards the heart. This helps stimulate the skin and the lymphatics and supports the large intestine during the elimination process.

Hot and cold showers

Start with a hot shower for two minutes then switch to cold for two minutes. Switch back and forth a few times, staying at hot or cold for at least two minutes each time, to allow the blood to flush to or away from the skin. This is said to be a good anti-ageing tonic and can be done daily.

'Fish and chips' bath

During Cleanse week I recommend doing a 'fish and chips' bath daily (or whenever you bathe if not every day). Sadly this doesn't mean eating fish and chips in the bath! It is lovely and relaxing, however. All you do is put a handful of Epsom salt flakes and a cup of apple cider vinegar in your bath water.

Epsom salt is rich in both magnesium and sulphate making it a valuable way to relax muscular tension, help blood flow and improve insulin uptake. It is also thought to support the elimination of toxins making it helpful during the Fertile Cleanse. Magnesium is required in the manufacturing of

Abdominal massage

Use a base oil like almond oil, and add a couple of drops of essential oils if you wish. Do not do this in the luteal phase (see page 216) if there is any chance that you could be pregnant. The best time to do this is between Days 7–14 of your cycle to improve the blood flow to the ovaries and uterus.

1 Lie on your back in a comfortable position. Using the flat of your fingers, begin over your tummy button, moving your fingers in small clockwise circles.

2 Gradually spiral out in ever increasing circular movements.

3 Once you have relaxed the whole area you can start to go a little deeper. Concentrate on the acupressure points situated on the lower abdomen (see diagram). Use your fingertips to stimulate these points, gradually applying pressure until you are penetrating the pressure further into the body.

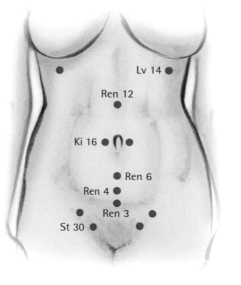

serotonin, a mood-elevating chemical produced in the gut and released in the brain giving a feeling of wellbeing and relaxation.

Cider vinegar is a good source of B vitamins and vitamin C so acts as a good skin tonic. Since the skin is also an organ of elimination it is important to nourish it during the Fertile Cleanse. It also helps kill bacteria and fungus, which can cause skin complaints.

Acupuncture

Acupuncture helps the function of the liver and also the large intestine. If you already have acupuncture tell your therapist if you are doing a Cleanse. Acupuncture can help support all the changes that are happening and help your body adapt. It is also very good for managing minor ailments. Headaches, bloating and sleep problems are symptoms that you might experience.

Liver compress

Finish each day of the Cleanse with a liver compress, as follows. At night fill a hot-water bottle with hot water. Dampen a towel with lukewarm water and squeeze out the excess. Wrap the towel around the hot-water bottle and sleep with the hot-water bottle on your liver (right ribcage).

Exercise during the Cleanse

Movement and moderate activity is very important during the Fertile Cleanse. But it is really a matter of regularity and not intensity. Many of us have very sedentary lives and sit at a desk, not getting out and about.

During the Cleanse focus more on doing something gentle every day; make it something you enjoy and can easily fit into your day. Walking in nature, getting off the tube or bus one stop earlier, dancing, yoga, a short jog around the block or a bicycle ride are all very beneficial to health and will not exhaust your Qi (energy). Twenty minutes of walking every day is beneficial.

Many people report the emotional benefits of exercise, which of course are a great side effect. However, watch that there is not an addictive element creeping in here. If you are using exercise to avoid emotional pain, this may not be the best way of dealing with your issues. Just as with food, be mindful about the reasons why you exercise and make sure you are honest about what you want to achieve. You may want a baby but the mind is complex and you may also desire a flat tummy or a red-carpet body. These goals are often incompatible with one another. So keep your eye on the main goal, which is a baby – in which case a flat tummy will joyfully be a thing of the past (for a little while).

Sleep

Getting a good night's sleep is very important for health and fertility, particularly when you are doing the Fertile Cleanse. Eating a light meal early in the evening will help the quality of your sleep, ensuring that your hormones become more balanced. When we sleep we produce growth hormone and melatonin, which are essential to allowing our body to repair. So think of night-time as for resting and repairing (and not digesting).

It is also our time to dream and to digest the day. The quality of our sleep can also be improved by not taking in too much additional information just before bed. Watching the news, working and surfing the internet before bed can all impact on the quality of our sleep. Give yourself a curfew on your digital time in the evening and try and keep it to a minimum. Perhaps during the Cleanse ban certain non-essential activities and give yourself some proper downtime.

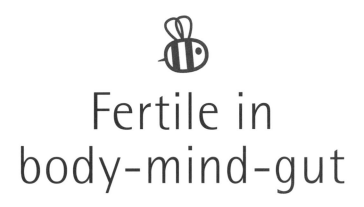

Fertile in body-mind-gut

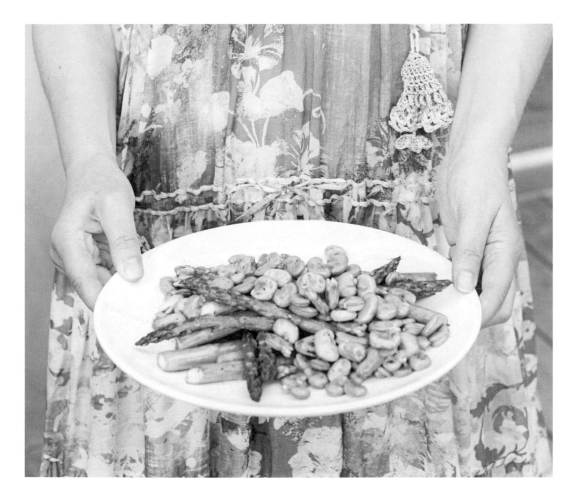

After years of observing and working with women (and men) trying to conceive I have concluded that many have poor digestive function. This is certainly not exclusive to fertility patients and, I imagine, it is very common in the wider population. Interestingly, it is often people who think they have a 'healthy' diet who tend to have the worst digestion. Modern living is often not conducive to creating a good digestion. Lack of time set aside for meal times, eating at our desk, eating late in the evening, leaving very little time to digest before bed, eating while stressed, flooding the digestive system with water, not chewing your food, too much fruit, raw food, juices, processed foods and consuming too many anti-nutrients all take their toll on our digestive systems.

There has been so much interest in diet in the past decade and this has resulted in a great deal of information on what constitutes a 'healthy' diet. But much of this advice is generic and does not consider the individual, or it is overly restrictive and leads to a very limited diet. This tends to create issues with the digestion as the diet is either not suitable for the person or it lacks variety. Another observation is that it tends to be the people who claim to have a 'healthy' diet who tend to have the least healthy relationship with food.

As well as making dietary changes, it is often important to address how and why we eat in the way we do. Together, nutritionist Victoria Wells and I have devised a programme using diet and acupuncture to support our patients' body, mind and gut. It has been a huge success and has helped improve the fertility and vitality of many men and women. In this chapter we have adapted the programme for you to do at home.

I recommend the Body-Mind-Gut Programme for patients who have suffered from any of the following issues:
• Digestive complaints: irritable bowel syndrome, allergies, intolerances.
• Chronic constipation.
• A history of weight issues.
• A history of yo-yo dieting.
• Thyroid issues.
• Immune issues: lowered immunity or those diagnosed with elevated natural killer cells.
• A history of autoimmune disorders (either personally or a strong family history).
• Endometriosis, polycystic ovary syndrome, Asherman's syndrome, fibroids.
• Repeated failed IVF cycles despite good embryo quality.

My body is a temple
Think of your body as a beautiful temple that has fallen into slight disrepair. The guttering is leaking a little and the dampness is seeping into the walls. As you look around this once gleaming place you see signs that the impact of the leak is becoming obvious in adjacent rooms.

Healthy gut facts

- Our guts are teeming with microorganisms. It's estimated that there are 40–100 trillion microbes in this inner ecosystem, with 1,200 species and they weigh about 2 kg. Our personal microbiota is as unique as our fingerprint.
- In poor gut health, zinc is one of the first nutrients our body has trouble absorbing.
- Your mouth is the 'gateway to the gut' – it is the first part of digestion. Your mouth can reflect the state of your digestion. Bad breath, gum disease and dental issues may all have their roots in poor gut health. Visit your dentist regularly and floss!
- A primal connection exists between our brain and our gut. We often talk about a 'gut feeling' and 'food for thought'. Most of the body's serotonin, an estimated 80–90 per cent of the total, is synthesised and stored in the gut; serotonin synthesis is regulated by gut microbes. Serotonin affects mood and social behaviour, appetite and digestion, sleep, memory and both sexual desire and sexual function.
- The small intestine is where the main digestive process occurs; breaking food down into tiny pieces. Food intolerances and allergies begin in the small intestine. If protein is not successfully broken down into amino acids, tiny particles enter the lymphatic system and confuse the immune system, contributing to allergy and intolerance.
- Women's hormones impact on the function of the large intestine, which is why your bowel movements may change throughout your cycle.

You decide it is time to do some repairs, so you go about stripping wallpaper away and spend hours deliberating over what beautiful new decorations you are going to use to return the temple to its former glory. You hire experts to hang the wallpaper so that you get the best finish you can. But after several months the problem reoccurs. Your beautiful new wallpaper has become uneven and is damp and discoloured in places.

You call in another expert who explains that this is a problem with the drainage and until you fix the guttering the problems will persist. No matter how beautiful you make the temple with wallpaper and paint, unless you deal with the origins of the problem you will just have to keep papering.

It is the same with the gut; so many people try to overhaul their diets, following programmes that do not support gut function and taking expensive vitamins, when actually they need to get their gut to function optimally. Once they have improved the health and microbes in the gut then and only then is it worth investing more widely.

Microbes

Gut microbes regulate digestion and metabolism, programme the immune system, maintain the integrity of the gut wall, influence the gut—brain connection and have a role in weight management.

Research in gut microbes is very exciting and we are starting to understand their influence on health and disease and the relevance to reproductive health.

Our gut microbes aid in the harvest of nutrients and in energy and nutrient formation from the food we eat. When the gut is out of balance the number of beneficial microbes is reduced and other microbes are able to increase their numbers. This is known as dysbiosis.

The main causes of intestinal dysbiosis are:

• Putrefaction (caused by diets high in fat and low in fibre).
• Fermentation (carbohydrate intolerance).
• Deficiency (caused by lack of dietary prebiotics or by antibiotic use).
• Sensitisation (abnormal immune responses).

The Body-Mind-Gut Programme

The Body-Mind-Gut Programme aims to heal and optimise gut health, improve nutritional status, mood and emotional wellbeing, and support fertility. After one month you will see improvements in your digestion, energy and emotional wellbeing. Longer term, the programme will help you choose and prepare foods that form a symbiotic diet – a diet that is rich in probiotic and prebiotic foods that support your microbiotia.

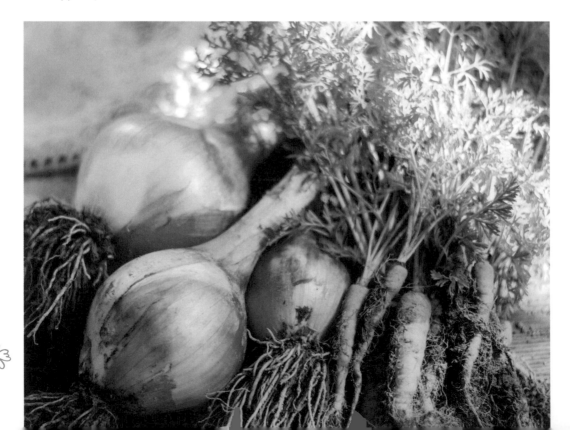

ASSESS: preparation

The first stage of the Body-Mind-Gut Programme is to assess yourself and identify any symptoms of gut dysbiosis.

Step 1

Use the self-assessment checklist and tick all the symptoms that apply to you.

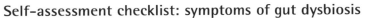

Self-assessment checklist: symptoms of gut dysbiosis

BOWEL MOVEMENT

☐ Irregular bowel movement

☐ Including intermittent or regular constipation or diarrhoea or both

☐ Undigested food in your stools

☐ Mucus in your stools

☐ Foul smelling stools or flatulence

☐ Feeling of incomplete evacuation

POST-EATING

☐ Abdominal pain

☐ Bloating after eating

☐ Excessive wind and/or burping

MOOD AND ENERGY

☐ Depression

☐ Anxiety

☐ Mood swings

☐ Fatigue

☐ Brain fog – lack of focus and clarity

☐ Poor memory

WEIGHT

☐ Difficulty losing excess weight

☐ Unexplained increase in weight

SKIN HEALTH – INFLAMMATORY OR ITCHY SKIN CONDITIONS

☐ Acne

☐ Eczema

☐ Hives

Step 2

Fill out the symptom tracker diary below to identify potential triggers and record your response to food. It is important to note that symptoms can occur the next day or even several days later so you need to be aware that symptoms may not be associated with the most recent food you have eaten. However, you may be able to identify patterns.

List any symptoms you are experiencing, including: pain or cramps; sudden urge to go to the toilet; loose stools or diarrhoea; constipation, straining and incomplete evacuation; excessive flatulence; nausea; bloating; mood swings; fatigue, tiredness or brain fog; anxiety or depression. Rate them on a scale of 1–10, as follows:

0	1	2	3	4	5	6	7	8	9	10
None	Mild	Mild	Mild	Moderate	Moderate	Strong	Strong	Strong	Severe	Severe

Symptom tracker diary

DAY	FOOD EATEN	SYMPTOMS	RATING
Monday			
Tuesday			
Wednesday			
Thursday			
Friday			
Saturday			
Sunday			

Step 3

I recommend making an appointment with a registered nutritionist to discuss your use of dietary supplements. You should take a 400-microgram folic acid tablet every day while you are trying to get pregnant and until you are 12 weeks pregnant. The Nurses' Health Study (*see page 79*) recommended the use of a multi-vitamin supplement for couples trying to conceive. The study found the risk of ovulatory infertility was lower among women who took a multi-vitamin supplement. Fertility supplements also contain the recommended dosage of folic acid and most contain vitamin D3.

Patients arrive in my clinic for their initial consultation reporting supplement use ranging from not taking the recommended folic acid to taking a wide range of supplements that in combination exceed the tolerable upper intake levels for individual nutrients. Some supplements, such as those in sachet, spray or liquid form, can be high in sugar and even artificial sweeteners. If you are taking certain medications, you need to avoid particular supplements. The body can very quickly re-establish balance when eating a diet rich in probiotic foods. However, it can be helpful to take a one-month course of probiotics to repopulate the gut.

CLEANSE: the first week

Start the programme by following the seven-day Fertile Cleanse (*see menu plan, pages 64–65*). The aim of the Cleanse is to remove from your diet sources of additives that contribute to gut dysbiosis, and to start to introduce a symbiotic diet.

The Body-Mind-Gut Programme has been devised to optimise gut health and to include foods beneficial for fertility. Unless there are special dietary considerations I do not recommend eliminating dairy or wholegrains as there is evidence from the Nurses' Health Study they may be important in the periconceptional period. I have discussed this in further detail below.

RESTORE: the second week

Restore gut health by introducing a symbiotic diet rich in prebiotic and probiotic foods. Follow the Body-Mind-Gut menu plan on pages 76–77.

Prebiotics stimulate growth or activity of beneficial microbes. Good sources include: wholegrains, bananas, onions, garlic, honey, artichokes and asparagus.

Cooking breaks down the fibre to some extent and some food sources are better at retaining fibre when cooked (such as onions, leeks and garlic – a sauce based on these ingredients is a good start to a symbiotic meal).

Polyphenols are a class of compounds found in plant foods that act as antioxidants and also as a food source for gut microbes. Ensure your diet includes a wide variety of vegetables, dark-coloured berries, nuts (particularly chestnut and hazelnut), seeds and fresh herbs and spices (add liberally to cooking, particularly cloves, star anise and oregano). Other sources include capers, olives and raw cacao.

Probiotics suppress and displace harmful microbes. There are many good reasons to introduce probiotic foods into your diet. Food sources include: natural yoghurt, kefir and fermented vegetables. Probiotic foods help maintain the right proportion of friendly bacteria needed for optimal health. One study found that people who consume fermented foods have less social anxiety.[1] Kefir, a live cultured milk drink made with dairy or coconut milk, is a good probiotic source to add to the diet and also meets the dairy recommendation of the Nurses' Health Study. Try to also get into the habit of serving sauerkraut or kimchi or other fermented vegetables with meals.

Body-Mind-Gut menu plan

DAY	BREAKFAST	LUNCH	DINNER	SUGGESTED SNACKS
1	Warm water with lemon *and* 'Carrot Cake' Overnight Oats (*see page 138*)	Aduki bean, Tomato & Miso Soup (*see page 148*)	Buckwheat Salad with Butternut Squash, Asparagus & Pecans (*see page 190*)	Beet Kvass (*see page 213*)
2	Warm water with lemon *and* Simple Overnight Oats (*see page 138*) with kefir pear, cinnamon, vanilla and almonds	Carrot, Sweet Potato & Coriander Soup (*see page 149*)	Almond-crusted Salmon with Cauliflower Purée (*see page 184*) served with Green Kraut (*see page 162*) **Vegetarian option:** Spiced Paneer with Wilted Greens (*see page 199*) served with Green Kraut (*see page 162*)	Avocado Kefir Lassi (*see page 211*)
3	Warm water with lemon *and* Mixed Grain Porridge with Blackberries, Hazelnuts & Flaxseeds (*see page 133*)	Beetroot Soup (*see page 144*)	Kidney Bean, Quinoa & Leek Salad with Toasted Pumpkin Seeds (*see page 195*)	Kefir Yoghurt Pot (*see page 211*)

DAY	BREAKFAST	LUNCH	DINNER	SUGGESTED SNACKS
4	Warm water with lemon *and* a poached egg with sautéed greens served with Green Kraut (*see page 162*)	Celeriac & Chestnut Soup with Chestnut & Herb Pesto (*see page 147*)	Beef, Broccoli & Quinoa Stir Fry (*see page 178*) **Vegetarian option:** Broccoli & Quinoa Stir Fry with Avocado & Toasted Cashews (*see page 198*)	Cannonball (any) (*see pages 209–210*)
5	Warm water with lemon *and* Quinoa, Chia Seed & Cardamom Porridge with Coconut, Pistachios & Raspberries (*see page 134*)	Leek & Fennel Soup with Toasted Walnuts (*see page 152*)	Beetroot & Coconut Curry (*see page 194*) served with Golden Kraut (*see page 161*) **Vegetarian option:** Dahl with Roasted Tomatoes (*see page 154*)	Probiotic Raspberry, Rose & Cardamom Jellies (*see page 208*)
6	Warm water with lemon *and* Baked Porridge with Goji Berries & Cinnamon (*see page 135*)	Grilled Mackerel with Probiotic Kohlrabi & Fennel Coleslaw (*see page 176*) **Vegetarian option:** Fragrant Aubergines (*see page 188*)	Dahl with Roasted Tomatoes (*see page 154*)	Kefir Yoghurt Pot (*see page 211*)
7	Warm water with lemon *and* an omelette with Lacto-fermented Salsa (*see page 164*)	Lentil & Leafy Greens Soup (*see page 157*)	Spiced Chicken Sauté with Leeks & Peppers (*see page 186*) **Vegetarian option:** Sweet Potato & Chickpea Gnocchi (*see page 200*) with Walnut & Rocket Pesto (*see page 166*)	Cannonball (any) (*see pages 209–210*)

INTEGRATE: a long-term eating plan

After two weeks following the menu plans, continue to eat a diet of natural foods. Avoid all processed foods. Eat well-sourced meat and fish, whole dairy, a wide variety of vegetables of different colours, a little fruit, bone broths, wholegrain, nuts and seeds. The key to a gut-friendly diet is variety. Any of the recipes in this book are suitable for the Body-Mind-Gut Programme, provided you introduce those that contain gluten slowly into your diet (*see opposite*).

- Eat bone broth daily.
- Include a probiotic dairy serving each day: try kefir or natural yoghurt.
- Increase your intake of fermented foods (*see box, opposite*).
- Don't eat highly processed refined foods or food containing artificial sweeteners, preservatives, emulsifiers and artificial flavourings (these alter gut microbes).
- Adopt practical strategies, being mindful when you eat away from the home.

Travelling and eating out

When you are away on holiday or travelling with work, or face periods when planning food is difficult, taking a probiotic supplement will help support your digestion. Eating out in restaurants can be difficult. Think about the sauces foods are cooked in and go for the options with the most natural ingredients. Choose plainer options with a good source of protein (fish or meat, grilled, steamed or baked) and plenty of side vegetables. Avoid breadcrumb-coated, crispy, gratin... And my best tip is: don't arrive hungry or cold. Otherwise you will be tempted by the hors-d'oeuvre and choose the most comforting (and possibly least healthy) dish on the menu.

Bone broths

A good bone broth provides flavour to dishes and nourishment for your body (*see page 142 for how to make it*). Broth is nutrient-dense, full of amino acids and minerals as well as collagen and cartilage. It has a long reputation as a traditional healing food and it may help with inflammation and digestive problems. The Body-Mind-Gut Programme uses bone broth in a daily soup and also as a warming drink. Hopefully drinking bone broth will become a daily habit. You can add flavours, including freshly grated turmeric, freshly grated ginger and chilli (*see page 142*), or make Beet Kvass (*see page 213*).

Reintroducing foods

As the gut heals, foods you may have eliminated may be tolerated better and reintroduced to the diet. For example, introduce grains containing gluten in small quantities. Choose grains that are more gentle on the digestive system, such as spelt, and use the symptom diary to track any gastro-intestinal response.

Dairy and kefir

The Nurses' Health Study was a major study that followed the diets of 18,000 women who were trying to get pregnant over a period of eight years. The study showed strong associations between diet and fertility and resulted in recommendations to improve fertility. The study indicated that a small amount of full-fat dairy may improve chances of becoming pregnant. The recommendation from the study was to aim for one to two servings of full-fat dairy products a day and to avoid any low-fat sources. For this reason, unless there are symptoms of dairy intolerance, sources of good quality dairy are recommended during the Body-Mind-Gut Programme.

Dairy kefir is probiotic and can usually be better tolerated by people who have symptoms of dairy intolerance as the fermentation process partially digests the milk proteins. It is a source of vitamins, minerals and essential acids and may play a role in calming inflammation and regulating immune function. Kefir made with whole milk meets the dairy recommendation from the Nurses' Health Study. Unsweetened probiotic kefir may take some getting used to — sweeten with a little raw honey (which is prebiotic) and gradually reduce the amount you add over time.

Wholegrains

Wholegrains are nourishing, warming and neutral in climate. The Nurses' Health Study found that choosing slowly digested carbohydrates that are rich in fibre can improve fertility. Wholegrains offer a good nutritional punch of prebiotic fibre, protein, fat, vitamins and minerals.

Serious gluten intolerance is seen in coeliac disease. This is an autoimmune disease where the reaction to gluten triggers a shrinking of the finger-like projections (villi) of the intestines' lining and sufferers become seriously ill after ingesting any amount of gluten.

The most common wholegrain foods contain gluten and many patients see an improvement in digestive symptoms, mood and energy levels when they eliminate these grains from their diet. This

Tips on including fermented foods

- Switch your normal bread to sourdough.
- Incorporate yoghurt into your meals; put a dollop of yoghurt into a bowl of vegetable soup and drizzle some cold-pressed oil on to dress it.
- Serve dill pickles as a condiment with meat and fish dishes.
- Serve kimchi or Naturally Fermented Sauerkraut (*see page 160*) as a condiment.
- Try Kombucha tea, a fermented drink that you make at home. It's quite fun and a little bit different. There is plenty of information online as to how to start.

may indicate gluten sensitivity but other factors that influence an improvement in health are the quantity and quality of wholegrain foods in the diet. Most people feel better when they cut down on excessive intake of processed bread, pasta and pizza! A wholegrain has three parts: the bran, the germ and the endosperm. To produce most of the flours, bread, cereals and pasta that we eat the grains are processed and refined by stripping out the bran and germ. These refined grains are less nutritious – losing 25 per cent of the grain's protein and other essential nutrients – and contain more gluten per unit of grain than wholegrains.

Gluten-free grains are permitted during the week one cleanse step of the Body-Mind-Gut Programme. These include: quinoa, gluten-free oats, buckwheat, rice, teff and amaranth. You can then slowly introduce a wider variety of wholegrains (use the symptom tracker).

If you are unable to reintroduce wholegrains to your diet this may indicate the need for testing. As coeliac disease has a significant genetic component, if anyone in your family has coeliac disease testing is recommended in any case. It is worth noting that miscarriages are common in women with untreated coeliac disease.

A fertile environment

'Are we becoming less fertile?' is a question I am constantly asked. It's also a question I constantly ask myself, and from my observations over 21 years in practice observing men's and women's fertility I would have to say that we are. When I speak to my medical colleagues who work in the field of fertility most will say that age is the single most significant feature in the decline in fertility in the individual. But I take a more holistic, even global view of what makes us fertile or not, and my observations are that women age at very different rates. Of course I am not denying the role age plays – that is a given – but I also believe that there are other factors at play, not least our environment.

Our environment has changed dramatically in the past decade and there is much speculation regarding global warming. Our food production has changed beyond recognition in the past 20 years. So has the sort of food we eat as well as the time we give over to buying, preparing and eating food.

Our bodies, too, have come under fire from a cocktail of chemicals that previous generations were not exposed to. We come into contact with low and high doses of these substances in many areas of our day-to-day life: in food, soil, air, water, household products, make-up products and in dentistry. These toxic substances may have a direct impact on our bodies and on our fertility and disrupt our immune system, hormonal systems and endocrine systems.

Exposure to environmental toxins can come from various sources and has been shown to have a negative impact on both male and female fertility. Bisphenol A (BPA), for example, found in plastic and food packaging, is an endocrine disruptor shown to decrease both sperm quality and sexual function, as well as being associated with chromosomally abnormal oocytes (egg cells) and recurrent miscarriage.[2] While oocytes are developing within the ovary they must withstand the impact of these substances in order to become competent and functional.[3] Air pollution, particularly nitrogen dioxide, has been implicated in reduced pregnancy rates and live births among women undergoing IVF.[4] Studies from the Czech Republic have demonstrated that men living in areas with high air pollution have a larger percentage of sperm that are morphologically abnormal with decreased motility and DNA fragmentation.[5] The Rubes study[6] is especially concerning, as it shows that DNA alone can be affected, while other sperm parameters remain normal; since few men are offered a DNA fragmentation test, this aspect of their fertility is often overlooked, with the result that their partners may be needlessly subjected to invasive treatments that are likely to fail.

Heavy metals, such as lead, mercury and cadmium, are present in the environment and enter the human body through contamination from food packaging, dental amalgams and consumption of larger fish such as tuna. While the benefits of eating oily fish may outweigh the dangers of exposure to mercury, care should be taken to consume smaller fish, which will reduce the exposure to heavy metals (*see page 40*).

There is some evidence that house plants may have the ability to absorb chemicals from the environment. NASA published a paper in the 1980s[7] investigating whether house plants used in enclosed space stations may have a role in reducing chemicals. They concluded that the following plants may be helpful: *Chlorophytum* (spider plant), *Dracaena* (dragon tree), *Scindapsus* (golden pothos) and *Hedera helix* (English ivy).

Bees, butterflies and other pollinators are facing extinction, which is bad news for us. When we see how nature is changing and how these creatures are struggling to survive and adapt to the evolving environment it is important to keep in mind that we are all part of the big cycle of life and we are not separate.

Our ability to receive nutrition

Two people can sit down to the same meal and, depending on their individual constitution and their attitude towards the food they are eating, they will absorb the nutrients in an entirely different way. I would go one step further and say that someone with a healthy attitude and a good relationship with food could eat a meal that wasn't nutritionally perfect yet absorb the nutrition very well, whereas a person with a poor digestion and an unhealthy attitude to the food will absorb the nutrients very badly. The bottom line is if we think a food will do us harm, it probably will – even if it's great food.

The way in which we receive nutrition depends on our ability to receive goodness and nourishment into our bodies. This belief comes from our early life experience of receiving love, nurture and nourishment. It can be interesting to observe your attitude towards food; observe when you reach for food and what you crave. Observe the impetus behind why you eat. Perhaps you are craving something else in your life: comfort, control, love, sweetness. Food can bring great nourishment and joy to people but you must be open to receive that nourishment and joy.

Planting seeds meditation

This meditation is an exercise to help focus your mind on nourishing and growing your ideas and visions. Do it every day when you are trying to bring something into your life. Instead of worrying about not being pregnant or if there is anything wrong, focus on the nourishment and germination of your ideas. Just like the bumblebee pollinates the garden, so impossible achievements spring from small beginnings.

- Lie or sit comfortably. Gently lay your right hand on the lower tummy over your womb and your left hand over your chest on your heart. Feel the connection between these two areas. Imagine the invisible connection, the energetic pull between the two centres. Enjoy this energetic pull, feel how the heart wants to communicate with the womb.
- Take a few moments to allow your body to relax, then bring your awareness to where your body meets the chair or bed, feeling the nature of that contact, that connection with the chair or bed.
- And then gradually become more aware of your body. You might become aware of some tension or tightness in an area of your body. Simply bring awareness to that area. Dissolve any tension. Dissolve any tightness through awareness.
- As you focus on your body, become more aware of the functions of your body.
- Allow yourself to become aware of your breath. Breathing in. And breathing out.
- Bring your awareness to your digestive system. Observe how your body naturally digests food.
- Be aware of your heart beating. How without effort your heart receives blood and then pumps it around the body.
- And simply be aware of all the cycles and rhythms of this amazing body.
- As you intuitively engage in the rhythms and cycles of your body, know that these resonate with the cycles of life, of the planet, of nature.
- Reflect upon the oceans ebbing and flowing.
- And the seasons coming and going.
- Reflect upon the fact that night is followed by day and day is followed by night.
- Reflect upon the cycle of the moon and the rising and setting of the sun.
- At this moment allow yourself to feel the fertile universe. Your fertile body. Everything in movement, everything in flow.

- And in a moment of your choosing take a deep breath.
- And on the out breath, fall into the centre of your body – into your solar plexus. And there I want you to imagine a very special garden.
- Imagine the soil is rich and fertile, full of bacteria and microbes, full of the nutrients of life all obeying the cycles and rhythms. Everything is in balance. Feel the deep rich colour of this soil.
- Imagine that you have with you a little bag of seeds.
- This is a time for planting your seeds in this fertile soil with intention and love, slowly and gracefully without haste or hurry. It is a time to plant the seeds in your own special garden for whatever it is you most wish for in your life.
- Have seeds for every conceivable outcome: seeds for a baby, seeds for love, seeds for happiness, for freedom, seeds for friendships, for loved ones, seeds for children, for parents, seeds for siblings.
- So scoop up a seed and create a clarity of intention. You and only you have access to this garden. You and only you know what is planted in your garden.
- When you have the clarity of intention, slowly, lovingly, gracefully plant this first seed deep into the soil of your garden, gently covering it over and blessing the seed.
- The seed knows how to flower with your intention, just as every acorn knows what it is to be an oak.
- Bless this seed and then reach into your sack for another seed and create an intention, a strong desire for what this seed will flower into in your life, in your loved ones' lives. Take a moment embedding this intention deep within this seed.
- And when you are ready, lovingly, gracefully plant this seed in rich, fertile soil, covering it like tucking in a small loved one at bedtime, blessing this seed.
- Feel the excitement at watching it grow in the days and weeks to come. And bid it farewell for this moment and return to your sack.
- Lift up a third seed and you and only you know what this seed will grow into, how this seed will manifest. Once again create a clarity of intention, imbue the seed with your heart's desire.
- Hold that focus and in your own time create a little hole in the soil, made especially for this third seed. And lovingly, tenderly cover the seed.
- Know that the cycle for this seed has already begun its journey through the darkness of the soil, bursting forth as a little shoot on its way to fulfilling its destiny. Think about why you wish to bring this into your life.

- Now turn back to your sack and take the next seed. Intuitively you know what it is you want to manifest from this seed. You and only you will know what it is you are creating in this lifetime.
- Your intention is strong. Your intention is powerful. It resonates with the oceans. It resonates with the night sky and the morning dawn.
- Take this seed and, with love and with great intent, plant it in your sacred garden. Bid it farewell on its cycle of evolution, of growing into that which it is meant to be.
- And now take your time to plant a few more seeds, taking loving care each time to create clarity and strength of intention.
- Lovingly remind each seed of its purpose in life: enjoying the fertility of the soil, enjoying being nourished by the earth, being connected to the earth and to heaven through the power of intention, being connected between the earth and heaven by the power of love.
- Each and every seed has its special place in the cycles and rhythms of our universe.
- Once you have completed your planting for today, take a moment to stand back and admire your handiwork.
- Hold in your mind each and every one of these seeds, feeling the excitement, the thought of them growing into shoots and beyond.
- Take a moment to water them in. Just sprinkle water over the earth, creating moisture.
- Bless all these seeds, and make a commitment to yourself to visit this secret garden each day – maybe even two or three times a day – to watch the growth of these seeds, to watch the little sprouts coming up from the earth, and to water your garden with love, with faith, with confidence in the ability of these seeds to reach their destiny.
- And as each seed flowers you will have a greater sense of your own destiny, your evolutionary cycle in this lifetime, who you came to be, what you came to do.
- Take a moment to feel the energy of gratitude, thankfulness for this sacred garden, for the seeds you have planted, for what will come to be.
- As you return to your daily life, know that your garden is fertile. Know that your garden is well nourished. Know that what is planted will grow to fruition.
- And honour yourself. Honour yourself as a tender gardener, planting your heart's desires and trusting their growth.
- Shanti, shanti, shanti.

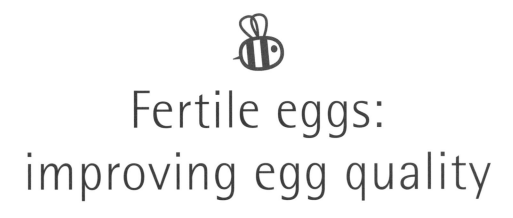

Fertile eggs: improving egg quality

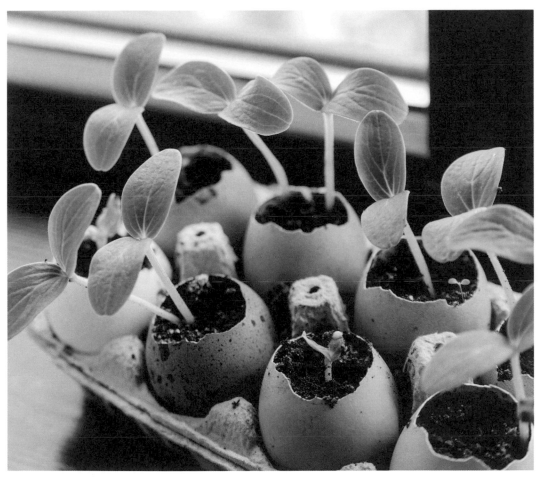

The age at which couples decide to start trying for a family is currently rising year on year, with one in 25 babies now being born to women over 40.[1] In 2013 nearly half (49 per cent) of all babies were born to women over 30, and 65 per cent to men aged 30 or over. The average age of first time mothers has risen to 29.8 compared with 26.4 in 1973.[1] Fertility declines with age; female fertility peaks in a woman's twenties and begins to decline more rapidly from around age 35.[2] At age 30, a woman's chance of conceiving each month is 20 per cent, and at age 40 this reduces to just five per cent.[3] Women are born with all the eggs they will have in their lifetime, and this number decreases with age, as each month an egg is released regardless of whether you are trying to get pregnant or not. Life is not perfect and it is not always possible to have our babies young, so many women find they are in the position of needing to discover ways to improve their egg quality. Egg quality is a hot issue and among the fertility community there is much discussion regarding how much can be done to slow down the ageing process or improve egg quality. My approach is to provide the body and the eggs with the right nutrients to support embryo development and to avoid harmful substances that speed up the ageing process.

Common thinking is that the quality of our eggs declines with age over time and at pretty much the same rate for everyone. I have a slightly different view, and although it is unlikely that we can turn back time or stay young for ever, small improvements in egg quality may be possible provided you create the right environment. The quality of our eggs is a combination of our genetic inheritance, the health of our mother while pregnant and our lifestyle (including diet and exposure to chemicals).

The eggs spend most of their time suspended in the ovaries and must go through a three- to four-month process called oocytogenesis. During this time they come under the influence of their environment and may be affected either negatively or positively. The other important phase is the follicular phase of the menstrual cycle (*the NOURISH phase, see page 48*). This phase gives a brief window where egg quality may be impacted on.

I have witnessed many times how making healthy changes to diet and lifestyle can improve IVF outcomes, increase pregnancy rates in those trying naturally and support women who have previously suffered miscarriage. It has always fascinated me that we are advised to avoid certain foods and toxins once we are pregnant, yet there is scant advice on this in the pre-pregnant stage. Yet those cells forming in your ovary may become your baby. They are full of life potential, so need to be nourished and preserved in just the same way as a baby in the womb would be.

Many pregnancies fail in the first few weeks after fertilisation, usually due to the quality of the egg. This may happen with or without the woman knowing she is pregnant. In natural conception it is thought that one-third of fertilised embryos become babies. In IVF it is likely that far fewer fertilised embryos become babies. These statistics largely come down to egg quality, which is the biggest factor determining whether an embryo survives or not as the egg helps determine the chromosomal status of the embryo. Many chromosomal issues occur in the period just prior to ovulation (the NOURISH phase) in the stage of development science calls meiosis. Meiosis has several phases: when we are embryos ourselves prior to birth; during the four-month period when the eggs are developing in the ovary; then finally in the follicular (NOURISH) phase of the menstrual cycle. When something goes wrong in any of the meiosis phases the incorrect number of chromosomes are created.

Mitochondria

Mitochondria are what give cells energy and power – they transform substances into energy that the cells can use, known as ATP. This is very like Qi in Chinese medicine. It is the motivating energetic force behind life and every biological process depends on it. The eggs are no different; they need a lot of ATP or Qi to grow and mature into a cell capable of becoming a baby. Over time, mitochondria can be damaged by toxins and oxidative stress, which may lead to chromosomal abnormalities. Equally, mitochondria (just like Qi) can be optimised by good nutrition, good blood flow (*see acupuncture and abdominal massage, page 67*) and a reduction in exposure to toxins, especially Bisphenol A (BPA).

BPA

Bisphenol A (BPA) is commonly found in plastic drink and food packaging and canned foods, as well as on cash-register receipts as a coating.

BPA is anti-oestrogenic; it reduces the amount of oestrogen produced by the ovaries. Other hormones critical to the developing follicles are also affected by BPA; these include testosterone, insulin and thyroid hormones.[4]

Animal studies have demonstrated that BPA exposure may cause chromosomal abnormalities in eggs and may also lead to hormonal imbalance. In 2012, a study into human fertility made a link between high levels of BPA and IVF failure and concluded that couples going through IVF should limit their exposure to BPA. The study has been repeated by Harvard researchers who found that

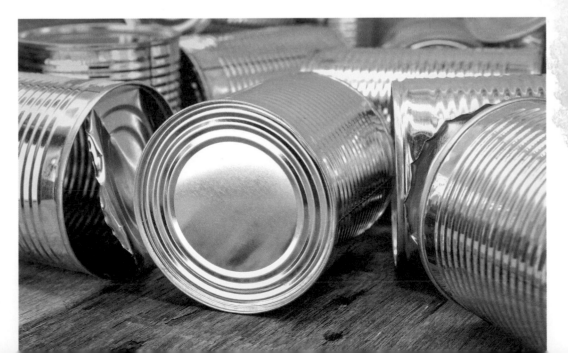

fewer embryos were produced during IVF in women with high levels of BPA and lower implantation rates were also found.[5]

IVF clinics rarely share this information with patients. Increased risk of miscarriage is also associated with BPA levels. The reason for this is not known but it may be due to chromosomal abnormalities. Levels of BPA have been found to be higher in women with polycystic ovary syndrome (*see page 97*) who often present with poor quality eggs.

Reducing exposure to BPA

Reducing exposure to BPA is relatively easy and inexpensive and is something that I advise all women to do no matter what their fertility situation. De-plastic your life, especially your kitchen. Replace plastic storage containers, bowls, cups and food-wrap with glass or ceramic. Takeaway plastic containers, ready-meal containers and coffee sachets may all contain BPA. It tends to be heating the plastic that releases the BPA; hot food, hot water and microwaves encourage the BPA to leak out of the plastic and into our food and drink. Use oven- or microwave-safe ceramic dishes instead.

Single-use plastic water and drink bottles tend not to contain BPA, although it is hard to be certain as products change all the time. Also, it's worth noting that products marked 'BPA-free' may not be as safe as you think. BPA-free products may contain BPA-related compounds as replacements that can have similar or even worse hormone-disrupting effects.

Phthalate

Another chemical found in many household and beauty products, including nail varnish and fragrances, phthalate is also thought to impact our hormones and fertility. Although these chemicals

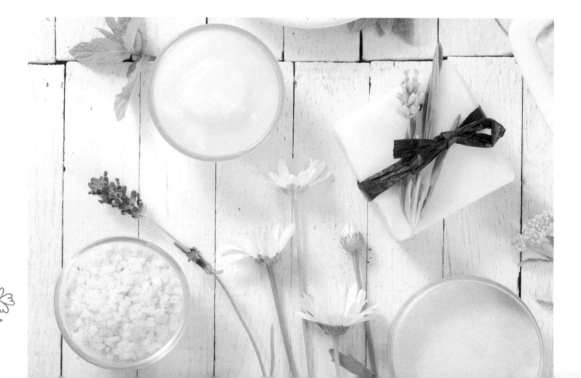

have been banned from children's products for many years, pregnant women and those trying to conceive are still frequently exposed to them.

Reducing exposure to phthalate

- Stop using nail varnish, at least for three to four months while you work on improving egg quality.
- Avoid beauty products that contain phthalates.
- If you see 'fragrance' on the label, avoid.
- Stop using scented candles in enclosed places.
- Don't use air fresheners.
- Switch to natural household products.
- Don't buy food wrapped in plastic, or remove it from the plastic wrapping as soon as you get it home.

Coenzyme Q_{10}

Coenzyme Q_{10} (CoQ_{10}) improves mitochondrial function and supplementation may have the potential to prevent or even reverse some of the decline in egg quality that comes with age. Your body synthesises CoQ_{10} but there are also food sources and it is available as a supplement. Beef, chicken and oily fish are good sources and nuts and seeds and some vegetables (including broccoli and cauliflower) provide smaller amounts. There is limited evidence, but little risk of side effects. I recommend using a supplement for its potential to improve egg quality in older women or women who are classified as 'poor responders' (please check with your physician). There are two forms of CoQ_{10} supplements and it is better to take the form of ubiquinol (as it is better absorbed than the other form, ubiquinone).

My approach

Where possible and when poor egg quality has been identified I would recommend a three- to four-month programme to improve egg quality before trying to conceive. Of course, this can be a tricky decision, especially for older women. But if it is possible it can bring great benefits. This long-term programme would include removing all potential chemicals from your environment and following the dietary recommendations for improving egg quality.

If you prefer to follow a short-term programme, aim to optimise health during the follicular phase. Refer to the NOURISH phase of the Menstrual Optimisation Plan (*see page 48*), and remove all chemicals from your environment.

If you are preparing for IVF, wherever possible follow the three- to four-month programme prior to starting IVF. If it is not possible, it is still worthwhile supporting an IVF cycle with the IVF Support menu plan (*see pages 119–120*) and also acupuncture where possible. Remove all chemicals from your environment. Of course, my aim is never to keep women from delaying and reducing their chances of success so age will determine how much time you can spend on preparing.

Nutrition to boost egg quality

- Balance your blood sugars (*see opposite*); give up sugar and refined carbohydrates.
- Take a good quality multi-vitamin, preferably for three to four months prior to conceiving.
- A high BMI (greater than 30) adversely affects egg quality and is associated with lower egg retrieval during IVF. (*See page 19 for tips on how to bring your BMI within the normal range*).
- Eat good quality protein (eggs, meat and fish).
- Consume healthy fats: oily fish, olive oil, avocados, nuts and seeds.
- Eat a wide range of different coloured vegetables and fruit to increase antioxidant intake to improve the ovarian environment and egg quality.
- Include foods rich in omega-3 fatty acids in your diet, such as oily fish (or supplement with marine plant omega-3 oil).
- Get plenty of vitamin D – from sunlight or as a supplement if you shown to be low in vitamin D from a blood test.

Melatonin

A hormone released during the night to regulate circadian rhythms, melatonin not only has a role in creating good quality sleep but is also important to fertility. An interesting fact is that high levels of melatonin are found in our follicles in the ovaries. It is thought that melatonin may have a protective mechanism for the ovaries and the developing eggs and act to protect the cells from damage by free radicals. Melatonin declines with age and this may expose the ovaries to more damage by free radicals and therefore more oxidative stress.

There is limited evidence suggesting that melatonin supplementation during IVF may improve egg and embryo quality for older women but more studies are required before melatonin supplementation can be recommended clinically. Furthermore, supplementation has been shown to interfere with ovulation so should not be used without advice from a physician. It should also not be used in conjunction with thyroid medication.

Get eight hours' sleep in a darkened room (make sure there is no light from streetlights or electrical equipment). Ensure that you sleep between similar hours every night to help maintain your melatonin levels. Spending a few hours outside in the daylight early in the day helps to boost your melatonin levels at night.

Drinking sour cherry juice has been shown to boost melatonin levels. Other food sources include: walnuts, tomatoes, grapes, peanuts and asparagus.

Balancing blood sugars

Eating regularly throughout the day keeps blood sugar and hormones in balance. When you miss meals the body can quickly kick into survival mode. I consider skipping meals as lost opportunities to consume healthy foods and it leaves you playing catch up for the rest of the day. Once you have that primal hunger or feel 'hangry' you crave more high-fat food and tend to over-eat, as the body feels deprived from the missed calories. If you are not a breakfast person, try at least to eat a small snack to kickstart your metabolism and break the fast.

Eating refined foods spikes your blood sugar and then it crashes, leaving you hungrier than before and reaching for the same foods again. Base your meals on vegetables with good protein sources to maintain blood sugar balance and add a serving of wholegrains.

DHEA

Dehydroepiandrosterone (DHEA) is a hormone precursor to testosterone and oestrogen. It is a produced by the adrenals and ovaries and DHEA levels usually decline with age. Supplementation of DHEA has been proposed to benefit women with diminished ovarian reserve by increasing egg quality and availability. Studies suggest that it increases spontaneous pregnancy rates[6] and improves IVF outcomes in poor responders with a history of failed IVF cycles[7]. However, other studies have suggested that DHEA supplementation does not enhance pregnancy outcomes in women with poor ovarian reserve[8] and that evidence-based recommendations for its use are lacking[9].

It is not clear which women benefit from supplementing with DHEA, although anecdotally women do report improvements. At the time of writing this book there is little compelling evidence to recommend DHEA supplementation for general subfertility. Women with polycystic ovary syndrome (PCOS) should not take DHEA as they already present with elevated androgens and supplementation may increase PCOS symptoms of acne and hirsutism. Women who have confirmed diminished reserves due to premature ovarian aging, poor responders to IVF and age-related infertility may benefit from DHEA supplementation.

Jing

I have talked about Jing already but it is very important to revisit in this chapter since there is a direct correlation between Jing and egg quality. Jing is a big deal in China; protecting and cultivating Jing is a national pastime! Like our reproductive capabilities, our Jing declines with age. It is our vital energy, creator of life. Our Jing is made up of two aspects: prenatal Jing, which is inherited from our parents and postnatal Jing, which is formed after birth through the food we eat and how we live our life. To

Foods to increase Jing

- Walnuts, almonds and pistachio nuts.
- Bone marrow, bone broth, chicken, kidney and liver.
- Artichokes.
- Mackerel, clams, mussels, scallops, oysters.
- Eggs.
- Sesame seeds.
- Seaweeds.
- Teas: nettle and rose hip.
- Supplements: chlorella and other micro-algae, royal jelly.
- Good quality full-fat milk (interestingly, this corresponds to the findings of the Nurses' Study – *see page 79*).

be abundant in Jing is to be fertile in body and mind, to inherit good reproductive capabilities and to have cultivated good health through balanced living and eating.

We deplete our Jing by burning the candle at both ends, overworking, trauma, excessive sexual activity, taking drugs, not recovering well after illness, emotional stress and poor lifestyle choices.

The quality of our Jing is reflected in the quality of either our eggs or, for men, the sperm. Someone in good Jing will possess strong reproductive energy, will be resilient to illness, robust in body and calm in mind.

The foods listed above are really powerful Jing foods and well worth including in the diet to improve egg quality.

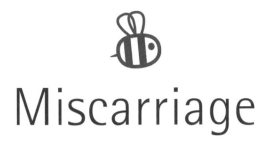

Miscarriage

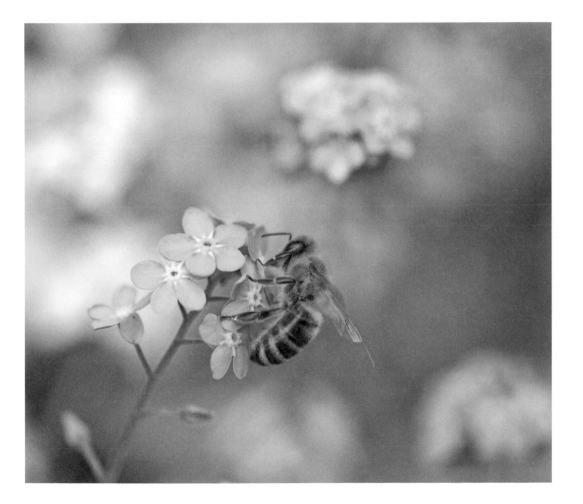

I sometimes ask myself if miscarriage is the last taboo. Certainly there is a great deal of denial about the suffering that it causes.

Of course, the reality is that there are not always answers, but sometimes that is because physicians lack the diagnostic tests and skills to help patients find an appropriate way forward. All too often the history of the patient is overlooked and they are fast tracked to IVF when the actual issue is miscarriage and not conception.

Taking a full history is vital. So often this reveals to me a pattern, be it from the family history or the patient's history. Anyone going through miscarriages needs to make sure they work with physicians who take a thorough history and don't ignore the facts.

There are so many different causes of miscarriage that many of them are beyond the scope of this book and they mostly cannot be fixed by diet alone. I have outlined all the possible known causes below and also given you some tips on recovery.

Coping with miscarriage

Following a miscarriage rest well and let yourself have time to recover. During the bleed include foods that move and activate Stagnant Blood (*see page 37*). This will encourage all the tissue to be expelled from the body. When the bleeding stops follow the guidelines for nourishing Blood (*see page 33*). When you get your first period follow the Menstrual Tonic (*see pages 52–54*).

Self-healing exercise

Set aside some time each day to focus on yourself and acknowledge how you are feeling. The purpose of this exercise is not to dwell; acknowledgment is a very different process where you are tending to your needs. Going within and building on your resources is a very empowering way of working with emotional wounds.

1 Instead of dwelling on the pain, think of things that make you feel good.

2 Now imagine the sensations; so, for example, if you feel good walking in the sun, ask yourself, 'Where do I feel this in my body?' If you feel it in your heart, investigate how that feels from there.

3 Use your imagination to expand on these feel-good feelings. Let them radiate through your body and let the energy of them penetrate into your whole being.

If the bleeding is prolonged and painful go back to your GP. I recommend that once the bleeding has stopped you have a scan to make sure that everything has returned to normal. This may not be offered as a free service and you may have to pay for a private scan. Or you can wait until the next period; if this is normal this probably means that everything is fine.

Emotions following a miscarriage can be changeable. It can be a very isolating experience and friends and family, with the best will in the world, often do not understand the suffering. Give yourself time to come to terms with the loss and to grieve. The temptation is often to rush into another pregnancy to try and fill the void.

When to start trying again? Miscarriage is energetically extremely draining, yet women recovering from miscarriage are never advised to rest and recover. This is critical and although the temptation is just to 'get back to normal', time spent recuperating is vital. Where there is time, I believe that leaving several months before starting to try again brings great benefits in subsequent pregnancies. The time left between trying again will depend on the nature of the miscarriage. If the miscarriage was straightforward and early then a couple of cycles is probably OK in a robust woman. However, in the case of infection, second trimester miscarriage, retained products, heavy blood loss or multiple miscarriages, taking several cycles out to recover is preferable (even six months, age allowing).

Pregnancy following miscarriage

I recommend that women who have had a previous miscarriage avoid sexual intercourse in the first 12 weeks of pregnancy. Taking adequate rest and avoiding exercise is also preferable in pregnant women who have previously suffered from miscarriage. Avoiding heavy lifting is also advisable.

Nutrition

Nutritional advice for women who have suffered a miscarriage focuses on factors that are associated with an increase in the risk of miscarriage, including weight, hormonal disorders, nutritional imbalances and immunological fertility issues, and also on supporting gut health.

There are nutrient deficiencies associated with miscarriage. Vitamin E deficiency has been associated with a higher rate of miscarriage. A study published in 2014 in the *American Journal of Clinical Nutrition* found that women with low levels of vitamin E are nearly twice as likely to have a miscarriage as those with adequate

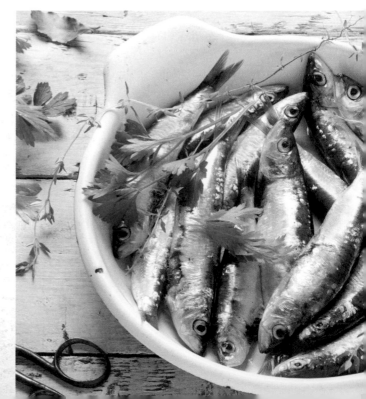

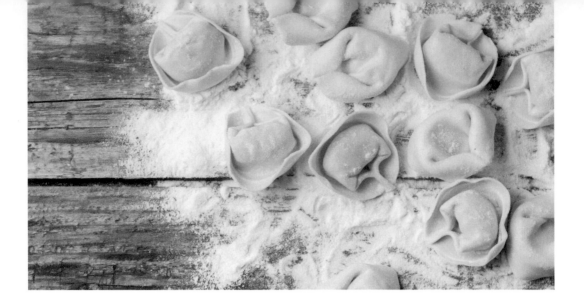

levels of the vitamin in their blood. Many women in the UK have low selenium status and selenium is important in pregnancy as an antioxidant. Several studies have investigated a possible link between low maternal selenium status and increased risk of miscarriage; however, the studies have been small and evidence is limited. The best dietary source of selenium is brazil nuts and other food sources are eggs, sunflower seeds, sardines and meat.

Gluten

Gluten is found in wheat, barley, oats, rye and corn. Wheat gluten contains alpha-gliadins (proteins) that trigger autoimmune coeliac disease in about one per cent of the population. They may also trigger inflammatory changes in non-coeliac patients. Any patient who has been diagnosed with autoimmune disease or elevated natural killer cells may benefit from removing gluten from their diet. If you have elevated immune markers there must be something triggering this. It could be environmental factors or stress, but often it is gluten. It is also worth looking at family history and identifying if there is a strong autoimmune tendency; if there is, experiment with cutting out gluten. There may be other foods but in my experience gluten is the most common. This gives an opportunity for the immune system to calm down and for the body to heal. As mentioned before, undiagnosed and untreated coeliac disease may contribute to recurrent pregnancy loss. Follow the Body-Mind-Gut Programme (*see pages 72–80*).

Causes of miscarriage

There are many reasons why a miscarriage may happen. The factors that may cause miscarriage include:
• Anatomical factors: uterine abnormality, fibroids, cervical incompetence.
• Hormonal factors: polycystic ovary syndrome, hormone 'deficiency', thyroid, prolactin.
• Chromosome abnormality.
• Immune mechanisms: NK cells, antiphospholipid antibodies, antinuclear antibodies, antithyroid antibodies, gliadin antibodies.

- Blood disorders (thrombophilias): factor V Leiden, protein C deficiency, protein S deficiency, antithrombin III deficiency, activated prothrombin C resistance (APCR), MTHFR C677T leading to hyperhomocytseinemia, G20210A prothrombin gene mutation, lupus anticoagulant, anti-cardiolipin antibodies.
- Infections and fever.

Anatomical factors

Congenital uterine abnormalities are more common in women with a history of repeated miscarriages. Congenital uterine abnormalities are also associated with preterm labour, fetal malpresentation and an increased risk of Caesarean delivery.

Congenital uterine abnormalities are usually picked up by HSG and can be evaluated more fully by 3D ultrasound imaging, hysteroscopy or MRI scan. The Royal College of Obstetricians and Gynaecologists recommends that all women with one or more second-trimester miscarriages should have their uterine cavity assessed using ultrasound. Any suspected abnormalities should be evaluated further using hysteroscopy, laparoscopy or 3D ultrasound.

Acquired uterine conditions

Although the existing evidence is inconclusive, certain acquired uterine conditions such as adhesions, Asherman's syndrome, fibroids and polyps have been suggested to increase the risk of pregnancy loss.

Hormonal factors

A percentage of pregnancies fail due to hormonal factors.

Polycystic ovary syndrome (PCOS)

This condition can cause infertility and frequently affects success of even conceiving. This syndrome together with a raised level of luteinising hormone (LH) results in an increased risk of miscarriage.

Hormone 'deficiency'

In pregnancies ending in miscarriage sometimes the levels of a hormone called progesterone are found to be low. This is thought to be the result rather than the cause of the miscarriage. Progesterone supplements do not appear to increase the likelihood of an ongoing pregnancy.

Thyroid

Hypothyroidism (underactive thyroid) has been linked to miscarriages during all trimesters. In the *Journal of Medical Screening* (September 2000) doctors reported that, by screening for thyroid problems before and during pregnancy, miscarriages could be reduced. Women with hypothyroidism have four times the risk of a second-trimester miscarriage.

Doctors look at the body's TSH levels to diagnose hypothyroidism, and a range of 0.3–3 is considered by many experts to be normal in sufferers. Some endocrinologists believe that a percentage of women may find it difficult to get pregnant, or maintain a pregnancy, at a TSH level above 2.0. This is one condition that is best treated with thyroid hormone medication. The medications used in hypothyroidism are safe to be taken during pregnancy. If you are prescribed Levothyroxine it should be taken on an empty stomach 30-60 minutes before food intake in the morning. This is to avoid erratic absorption of the hormone.

Hypothyroidism can affect fertility in the following ways: disrupting ovulation, shortening the luteal phase, oestrogen dominance, progesterone deficiency. Commonly reported symptoms of hypothyroidism include: exhaustion, weight gain, dryness of hair, nails and skin, loss of libido, sensitivity to cold and difficulty getting warm, mood swings.

Hyperthyroidism (overactive thyroid) can affect fertility by disrupting the menstrual cycle, leading to irregular or absent periods. This in turn can affect ovulation. Common symptoms and signs of an overactive thyroid include: hyperactivity, mood swings, insomnia, feeling tired all the time, feeling weak, sensitivity to heat and excess sweating, unexplained weight loss, needing to pass urine or stools often, irregular periods, irregular or fast heart rate, tremor or shake/twitch.

Prolactin

Prolactin is a hormone secreted by the corpus luteum of the ovary that may affect ovulation. High levels of prolactin can also affect the function of the ovaries by interfering with the hormones that control these glands. In women, this can lead to irregularity (oligomenorrhoea) or even a complete stopping of menstrual periods (amenorrhoea), reduced fertility and menopausal symptoms, like hot flushes.

Chromosome abnormality

Chromosomal analysis involves taking a blood test from both the man and the woman and sending the samples to a genetics laboratory. The results can take between four and six weeks to obtain.

There is no treatment that can alter the chromosomes in an individual if they are already abnormal. If the analysis shows that you or your partner carries an abnormality, then you will be offered specialist genetic counselling to give you more information and help you decide about future pregnancies.

Your clinic may offer to carry out chromosomal analysis of fetal tissue, although this can depend on the laboratory facilities available. It involves sending tissue from the miscarriage to the genetics laboratory where it undergoes the same process as for blood. Unfortunately a result is obtained only in approximately half of cases. It takes about six to eight weeks or more to obtain the results. If the result is abnormal, but both parents have a normal chromosome pattern, then the abnormality in the baby is unlikely to recur in a subsequent pregnancy.

Blood disorders (thrombophilias)

The thrombophilias are a group of disorders that promotes blood clotting. Individuals with a thrombophilia tend to form blood clots too easily, either because their bodies make too much of certain proteins, called blood-clotting factors, or too little of anti-clotting proteins that limit clot formation. As many as one in five people in this country has a thrombophilia.

Most people with a thrombophilia do not know they have it because they have no symptoms. However, some will develop a blood clot where it does not belong. Often, blood clots form in the lower leg, causing swelling, redness and discomfort. This condition, called deep vein thrombosis, is often diagnosed with ultrasound or other imaging tests.

Pregnancy is another time when signs of thrombophilia are more common. Most women with a thrombophilia have healthy pregnancies. The thrombophilias may, however, also cause a severe form of pre-eclampsia, a pregnancy-related disorder that can pose serious risks for mother and baby, which is characterised by high blood pressure and protein in the urine. Most of these problems are believed to result from blood clots in placental blood vessels that lead to placenta changes and reduced blood flow to the fetus.

If you have a blood disorder, you will be offered a combination of low-dose aspirin plus low-molecular weight heparin injections. This will dramatically reduce the risk of miscarriage and gives you an excellent chance of a successful outcome. The therapy may need to be started before pregnancy occurs, and continued four to six weeks after birth. If your results revealed that you are a carrier of MTHFR gene mutation, you will be offered folic acid supplementation of 800mcg/day.

Infections and fever

Fever at the time of ovulation can disturb cell division and can lead to chromosomal abnormalities and miscarriage. High fever in pregnancy is usually managed effectively with paracetamol and lots of fluids and bed rest.

Sometimes infections are already present in the endometrium before conception, such as endometriosis, and the inflammation they cause can irritate the fetal membranes and cause premature contractions of the uterus.

Other infections

German measles (rubella), chicken pox (herpes zoster), the genital herpes virus (herpes simplex), syphilis and tuberculosis, and parasites such as those causing toxoplasmosis and malaria can all affect the fetus. If the damage to the fetus is serious, then it will miscarry. Sadly, in some cases of rubella and syphilis infection the baby will survive but be born with serious abnormalities.

Infections in the genitourinary tract active at the time of pregnancy increase the risk of second-trimester miscarriage about threefold over normal.

Other possible causes of miscarriage

In Chinese medicine, the following are also considered possible causes of miscarriage.

Accidents

Accidents such as serious falls or shocks are sometimes blamed for miscarriages. Falls and injuries can cause Blood to Stagnate, which may manifest as a disorder of blood flow in the placenta or endometrium. Shock can also affect the Heart energy by scattering it and impacting on the flow of Blood to the uterus and for the nourishment of the fetus.

Heavy lifting

Strain of the lower back associated with lifting heavy loads can also cause a miscarriage. Studies have shown that work that involves lifting and bending can increase the risk of miscarriage more than threefold above normal.

Alcohol and drugs

Alcohol or drug abuse can create toxicity in the fetus that it cannot survive. In terms of the internal climate this is seen as internal Heat that can damage the endometrium and the blood.

Hot baths

The use of hot tubs is a risk for miscarriage, especially in the first few weeks of pregnancy. The regular use of bathtubs does not seem to be a risk factor, but sustained elevation of core body temperature is best avoided.

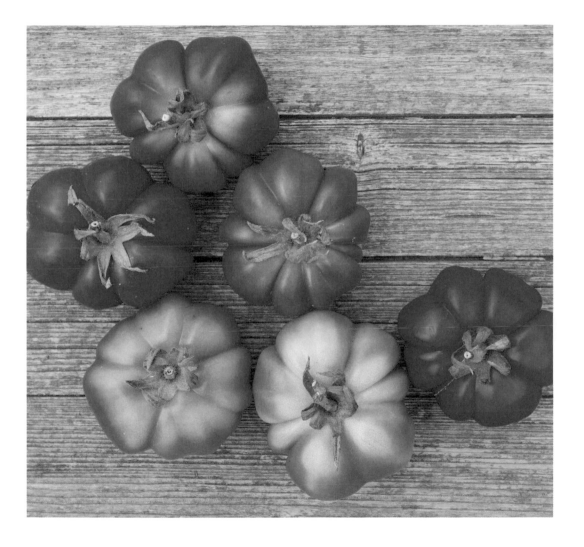

Fertile man

It is the health of both parents at the time of conception that determines the health of the child. All too often male fertility is overlooked, with all the attention being directed towards the female partner. But it is estimated that male factor fertility makes up 40 per cent of all infertility with a further 20 per cent of cases being due to mixed male/female factors.

Age does play a part in male fertility, but less dramatically than it does for women with the steady decline of egg quantity and quality. There is little by way of treatment offered to men by mainstream medicine in terms of improving quality of sperm, so diet and lifestyle changes offer the best chance for men to optimise and preserve fertility.

There is anecdotal evidence that male infertility is on the increase. Certainly, my observations are that semen samples contain a higher percentage of abnormal forms than they did ten years ago. Female fertility awareness has really improved, but there is still a lack of awareness among men and also a lack of acknowledgement from some medical professions of the importance of male fertility. In part this problem comes from the fact that fertility specialists tend to be gynaecologists, in other words specialists in female reproduction.

Although this is a chapter on male fertility I am not keen that everyone eats different foods – I feel that this would be counterproductive and not achieve the desired results. I want you to let go of control around food and spending too much time worrying about it. Instead I want you to learn to tweak dishes to suit the individual. A sprinkle of super seeds there, a dollop of soured cream, a drizzle of oil – each of these additions for the right person can make a difference. It's the small things.

General advice

Diet and lifestyle play important roles in male health and fertility. There is evidence that specific nutrients support fertility. Good sperm health includes count, morphology (structure) and motility (movement). There also needs to be good levels of semen to transport and provide energy for the

Fascinating facts about sperm

- Men produce sperm continually.
- It takes three months to produce sperm and this is called spermatogenesis.
- Sperm can survive inside the female for 48 hours but I have known it to survive for 5 days.
- 300 million sperm per day mature every day.
- Sperm do not like heat.

sperm. It is generally said that sperm takes 90 days to mature but actually it is closer to two and a half months. Sperm develop in the testicles for 50-60 days and are then excreted into the sperm-maturing tube, the epididymis, to complete their maturation for another 14 days.

Soya can disturb hormonal balance in both men and women through its high phytoestrogen content (*see page 41*). One study in 2008 found that a high intake of soya foods in male diets was associated with lower sperm concentration.[1]

Men need to maintain a healthy weight and take regular exercise. It is advised to reduce alcohol and caffeine intake and refrain from smoking. It is clear that smoking negatively affects sperm concentration, motility, and the proportion of normal sperm as well as impacting negatively on the genetics of sperm. An observational study of the alcohol intake of 1,221 Danish military recruits published in *The BMJ*[2] suggests that moderate alcohol intake of at least five units every week is linked to poorer sperm quality.

Heat

Heat is a significant problem for sperm. Male chefs, for example, have a high incidence of infertility since their testicles are exposed to a constant heat source.[3] Keep the testicles cool by wearing loose-fitting boxer shorts to avoid over-heating. A study found that tight-fitting underwear created a 50 per cent reduction in semen parameters (count, morphology and motility).[4]

Working out in hot rooms or a prolonged rise in body temperature, particularly locally to the testicles, is not good for sperm. Men who cycle long distances may damage their fertility due to heat build-up and local trauma. It is also possible that mobile phones carried near to the testicles, or heated car seats may impact on sperm and using laptops connected wirelessly to the internet directly on the lap may also decrease male fertility.[5, 6]

Varicoceles

Varicoceles are varicose-like veins that affect the small veins around the testicles. They are more common in men with fertility problems than the general population; the evidence of the benefit of removing them is varied, especially for fertility purposes alone. However, if diagnosed at a young age the possible detrimental effect of a long period of high testicular temperatures over many years may justify the removal of them as a preventative measure. Following the Blood Stagnation and Damp diet can be of benefit if you have varicoceles.

Thyroid health and male fertility

Thyroid function can impact on sexual performance, erectile dysfunction, low libido and premature ejaculation. Hypothyroidism (underactive thyroid) can affect morphology and hyperthyroidism (over-active thyroid) can affect motility.

Weight

A BMI of 19–24 is ideal for male fertility. Male BMI may also correlate with the outcome of fertility treatment, with a reduction in live birth rates from IVF correlating with increasing BMI and a poorer embryo development rate. Yet, interestingly, IVF units rarely advise men on weight loss.

Male fertile tendencies

Men typically fall into one of the five tendencies below, or a combination of the tendencies, for example Damp-Heat or Damp-Cold. Read through the symptoms for each category to find out which one(s) you identify with. You won't necessarily have all the symptoms, so just focus on your main symptom or those that reoccur regularly. Once you've found your tendency, read the diet advice for each type in the Fertile Food chapter (*see pages 27–42*).

Hot tendency symptoms

Heat is not a good thing for sperm but mainstream medicine only considers external sources of heat as potentially causing injury to sperm. It is well documented that Jacuzzi's, steam rooms, tight boxer shorts, cycling, heated car seats and other forms of external heat may cause damage to sperm, yet there is no knowledge or understanding that Heat can be generated internally.

- You produce scant ejaculate.
- You are unable to maintain an erection.
- You produce scant urine that is dark yellow in colour.
- You are restless.
- You feel hot.
- You get agitated.
- You have abnormal sperm morphology (a high number of sperm with abnormal shape).
- Your tongue is red.

Stagnant (Qi) tendency symptoms

This tendency is usually underpinned by emotional swings, especially frustration and anger (or suppressed anger).

- You have pain or an uncomfortable sensation in your testicles.
- You are disinterested in sex or have a low libido.
- You suffer from low-level depression or experience mood swings.
- You feel disconnected to sex and to life in general.
- You sigh a lot.
- You are irritable.
- You have physical symptoms that come and go, especially digestive symptoms.

Damp tendency symptoms

- You have a history of sexually transmitted diseases.
- You suffer from genital itching.
- You feel that you body is heavy.
- You experience heaviness in your testicles.
- You have discharge, especially from the penis.
- Your ejaculate is yellow and cloudy.
- Your urine is cloudy.
- Your sperm is clumped.

Cold tendency symptoms

Warmth is needed to activate the production and release of sperm; think of it in terms of having 'fire in your belly'.

- You have a low libido.
- You have pain in your lower back.
- You have an abdomen that is cold to touch.
- You may have mild incontinence.

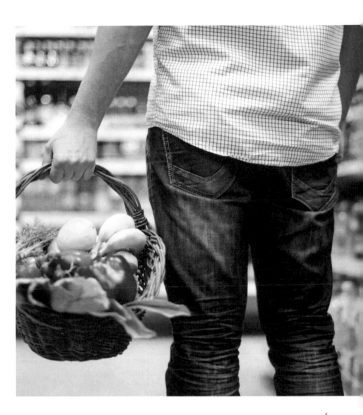

Blood Stagnant symptoms

- You have varicoceles (an abnormal distension of the veins in the spermatic cord of the scrotum).
- You have varicose veins.
- The colour of your testicles is purple.
- The colour of your tongue is purple.
- You suffer from pain that is fixed or sharp like a knife.

Key nutrients for healthy sperm

The male fertility diet does not differ much from a woman's fertility diet but there is evidence that specific nutrients can improve sperm function. The diet should include healthy fats, good sources of protein and a wide variety of colourful vegetables and fruit to provide vitamins, minerals, fibre and carotenoids and other phytochemicals. Eliminate processed foods and avoid artificial sweeteners, preservatives, emulsifiers and stabilisers and introduce probiotic and prebiotic foods. Eat organically where possible. The diet that is important for sperm health is also important for the long-term health and development of the child and ensures that Dad is around to raise his child too! And eating healthily will increase libido.

- **Carotenoids** may improve semen motility and lycopene (found in tomatoes) is associated with improved sperm morphology. Carotenoid-rich fruit and vegetables include: carrots, sweet potatoes, avocados, dark green leafy vegetables, cantaloupe melon, red peppers, tomatoes and dried apricots. One tip is to eat these vegetables when they have been cooked in oil or are dressed in oil as fat is required for absorption of the carotenoids in the intestines.
- **CoQ$_{10}$** is necessary for sperm motility, improves sperm health and protects from damage. Sources include: beef offal, chicken and oily fish, nuts and seeds. Some vegetables (including broccoli and cauliflower) provide smaller amounts.
- **Folate** boosts sperm health. Sources include: green leafy vegetables (broccoli, Brussels sprouts, spinach), asparagus, liver, chickpeas, brown rice.
- **L-arginine** increases sperm count, motility, quality and ejaculate volume. Sources of this amino acid include: red meat, nuts (almonds, walnuts, hazelnuts, cashews, peanuts), seafood, dairy products, chocolate.
- **L-carnitine** is necessary for normal sperm function – concentration and quality and motility. Good sources include: beef, pork and seafood.
- **Omega-3 long-chain fatty acids** improves sperm quality, motility and count. Semen is rich in the prostaglandins produced from omega-3 long-chain fatty acids. Omega-3 long-chain fatty acids are found in oily fish. Fish oil supplements may help improve the all-important ratio of omega-6 to omega-3 in the diet. Non-fish eaters can supplement with marine plant-based supplements. Plant sources, including walnuts, flaxseeds and chia seeds, provide short-chain fatty acids that have a limited conversion to long-chain fatty acids in the body.
- **Selenium** improves sperm count and protects from oxidative damage in developing sperm. Sources include: nuts and seeds (particularly brazil nuts and sunflower seeds), fish (mackerel, halibut, tuna, herring, sardines), shellfish (oysters, scallops, lobster), poultry, meat and wholegrains.

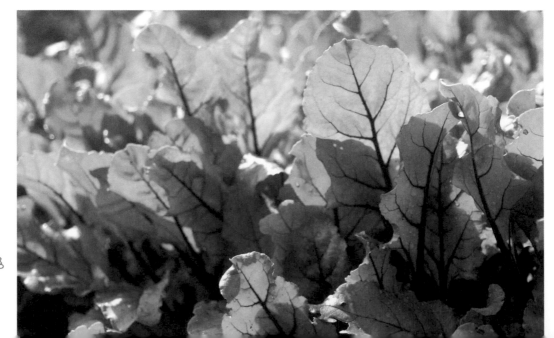

- **Vitamin B$_{12}$** is good for increasing sperm count and motility. Good sources include: fish, shellfish, dairy, offal, eggs, beef, pork.
- **Vitamin C** improves sperm structure and count, and protects against oxidative damage. It also plays a role in keeping sperm from clumping together thereby boosting sperm motility. Sources include: peppers, citrus fruits, berries, leafy green vegetables.
- **Vitamin D** helps maintain semen quality and sperm count and is necessary for healthy development of sperm. Sunshine, not food, is where most of your vitamin D comes from. To ensure adequate vitamin D status you need regular daily sun exposure (without sunscreen for a short period of time). Very few foods in nature contain vitamin D and you cannot meet needs with diet alone. A combination of diet plus sunlight may provide acceptable levels of this vitamin. The best dietary source is oily fish and, in lesser amounts, meat, eggs and milk. Fortified foods such as boxed break-fast cereals are not generally recommended as they tend to have low nutritional value generally. A vitamin D supplement may be advisable for men with darker skin tones and men who spend very little time outside during the summer.
- **Vitamin E** is an important antioxidant to help protect sperm and improves sperm health and motility. Sources include: sunflower seeds, almonds, spinach, Swiss chard, avocado, peanuts.
- **Zinc** increases sperm count, morphology and motility and contributes to normal DNA synthesis and protects from oxidative stress. The concentration of zinc in semen is high. Sources of zinc include: oysters, lentils, pumpkin seeds, nuts, spinach, chicken, lamb, pork and cocoa.

Recipes for boosting male fertility

- Almond-crusted Salmon with Cauliflower Purée (*see page 184*)
- Avocado Kefir Lassi (*see page 211*)
- Nut, Spice & Seed Mix (*see page 168*)
- Chickpea & Date Houmous (*see page 170*)
- Nourishing Coconut, Date & Almond Drink (*see page 212*)
- 'Carrot Cake' Overnight Oats (*see page 138*)
- Kefir Cheese-stuffed Peppers (*see box, page 163*)
- Walnut or Almond Tarator Sauce (*see page 165*)
- Walnut & Rocket Pesto (*see page 166*)
- Spicy Pumpkin Seeds (*see page 169*)
- Lacto-fermented Salsa (*see page 164*)
- Oyster, Leek & Sweet Potato Soup with Japanese 7-spice Powder (*see page 146*)
- Sardine Pâté (*see page 169*)
- Roasted Sardines with Tomato, Onion & Pomegranate (*see page 177*)
- Moroccan-spiced Chicken Livers (*see page 172*)
- Dahl with Roasted Tomatoes (*see page 154*)

Three foods to boost sperm health

Walnuts

- One study found that eating two hand-fuls of walnuts a day improved the shape, vitality and motility of sperm.[7]
- Walnut recipes: Walnut & Rocket Pesto (*see page 166*), Walnut-crusted Salmon (*see page 184*), Lemon Kefir Cheesecake (*see page 206*).
- Take to work: Walnut & Rocket Pesto (*see page 166*) on oatcakes, walnut and almond trail mix.

Pumpkin seeds

- Pumpkin seeds contain phytoesterols – these improve testosterone production and reduce the size of enlarged production.
- Pumpkin seed recipes: Nut, Spice & Seed Mix (*see page 168*), Amaranth, Spiced Pear & Pumpkin Seed Porridge (*see page 130*), Kidney Bean, Quinoa & Leek Salad with Toasted Pumpkin Seeds (*see page 195*).
- Take to work: Trail mix, Spicy Pumpkin Seeds (*see page 169*).

Tomatoes

- One of the best food sources of the carot-enoid lycopene, associated with improved sperm shape, count and viability.[8]
- Lycophene is better absorbed when eaten with dietary fat – olive oil or avocado.
- Tomato recipes: Omelette with Lacto-fermented Salsa (*see page 164*), Aduki Bean, Tomato & Miso Soup (*see page 148*), Dahl with Roasted Tomatoes (*see page 154*), Roasted Sardines with Tomato, Onion & Pomegranate (*see page 177*).
- Take to work: Sun-dried tomato pesto and oatcakes.

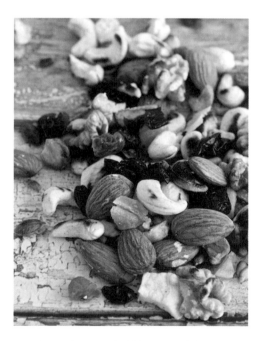

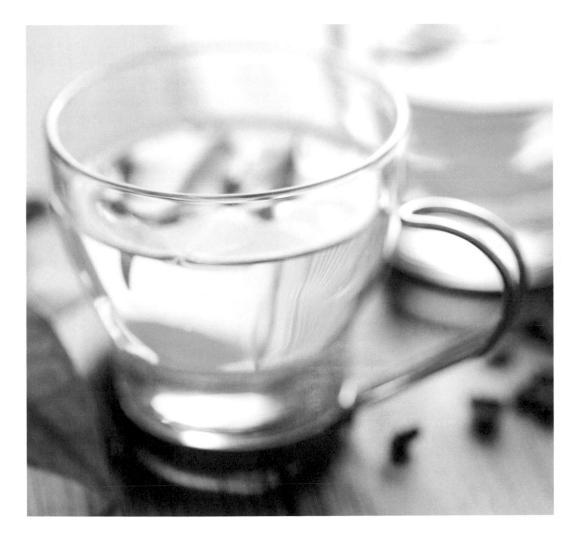

IVF support

Every year more couples seek assistance from assisted reproductive technologies (ART). A major part of what I do as a practitioner is to support couples through fertility treatment; giving the patient some fine-tuning with acupuncture, preparing them through good nutrition, helping the body and helping to create a calm mind.

Becoming parents through what can feel like a very clinical process can make even the most calm person feel like they are out of control. The process of going through IVF provides it own challenges to the body and emotions. There is much you can do to support that process through preparation and during IVF treatment itself. The supporting roles of good diet and a calm mind are just that, supporting. They are not the main event but can help you to feel grounded, healthy in your body and relaxed during this time.

I help a great number of women through IVF in my clinic and have discovered over the years that they love to engage in this process through the IVF store cupboard lists and recipes we provide. My IVF patients in particular will often ask me for extra recipes and what to eat and when during their cycles for maximum support. There are a number of common symptoms women experience during IVF that can be alleviated through nutrition and calming the mind along with the acupuncture I offer. These include bloating or constipation, difficulties with sleeping, tension headaches and anxiety.

Receiving support during IVF

Being offered support and allowing yourself to accept support are two very different things. Often the support is there on offer for us, but for one reason or another we find it hard to receive it. Notice how often someone offers you help and you reply with the words, 'Oh, I'm fine'. That may or may not be true; have an awareness of this and see if you catch yourself out.

It might be that there are lots of people who want to help you, but they aren't sure how. Sometimes at difficult times we end up being the teacher and showing people how we need to be supported. Then when the support is given it is very much up to us to allow ourselves to receive it. Sometimes this might feel like too much hard work; but actually allowing yourself to receive is a very fertile act of self-love. Of course, some couples find that they easily support one another in the right way and instinctively know what each other needs. This is wonderful and they are blessed; don't ever lose that as it is a precious thing. Other couples have different dynamics and have different reasons for being together. Many spiritual beliefs talk about the idea that we chose our partners because of the lessons we need to learn in life, from each other.

A relationship is like a mirror being held up to us constantly reinforcing the part of our personality or psyche that needs attention. Going through huge life-changing experiences gives us each an opportunity to learn and grow. It's hard to view IVF and the infertility struggle in this way and I do not mean to underplay the intensely emotional challenges it presents to couples. But it can offer you an opportunity to deepen your experience with life and with each other.

IVF explained

IVF involves collecting eggs from the female partner and sperm from the male partner or a donor/ anonymous donor, and bringing them together in laboratory conditions with the aim of fertilisation. If fertilisation takes place, the fertilised egg or embryo is returned to the uterus to implant.

The stages of IVF

There are four main stages of IVF: the stimulation phase, egg collection, fertilisation and embryo transfer.

1 Stimulation phase

You are given hormone drugs to stimulate your ovaries to produce multiple follicles and therefore multiple eggs for collection.

2 Egg collection

After 10–14 days of being given the stimulation drugs, you will be shown how to self-administer an injection of HCG (human chorionic gonadotropin), which encourages maturation of the eggs and easy release at time of collection, which will be 36 hours later. Egg collection usually takes place under deep sedation so that the process should be pain free.

3 Fertilisation

The eggs will then be mixed with the sperm for fertilisation to occur. If there are any problems with the sperm then ICSI (Intra-cytoplasmic sperm injection) will be needed to improve the fertilisation rate. ICSI is a treatment where a single sperm is injected directly into the egg and is mainly used when there is low sperm count or high sperm abnormality.

4 Embryo transfer

A fertilised egg (sometimes two or three) is transferred back into your uterus, usually three days after collection. You will be given progesterone at this stage to help with implantation. You may also be given aspirin, heparin or steroids.

'Long protocol' IVF

In 'long protocol' IVF you will be treated before the IVF cycle to down-regulate your hormones. Medication is given to put the body into a temporary state of menopause, in other words stopping the body's natural cycle. This is done to prevent any eggs being released too early for collection. This will usually last 10–14 days, after which you are scanned to check the medication worked and that your endometrium is a good thickness before moving to the stimulation phase.

Your IVF physician will decide which cycle is most appropriate.

The IVF cycle

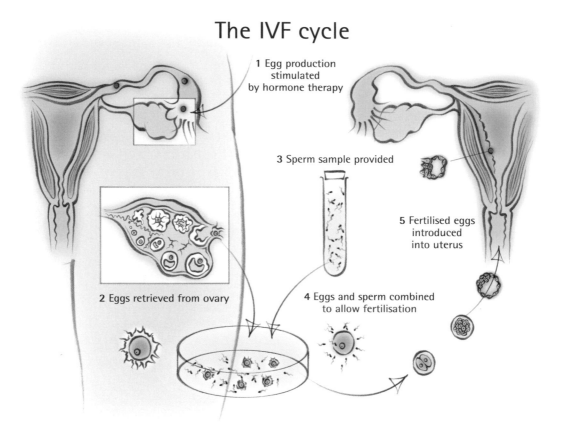

1 Egg production stimulated by hormone therapy

2 Eggs retrieved from ovary

3 Sperm sample provided

4 Eggs and sperm combined to allow fertilisation

5 Fertilised eggs introduced into uterus

'Natural IVF'

With 'natural IVF', minimal medication is used which means that you will only be likely to produce one or two eggs during the cycle. Success rates are lower but less medication is thought to be of possible benefit for women who are older and more likely to produce viable eggs in a natural cycle.

Egg freezing and embryo freezing

Egg freezing is when eggs are extracted from a woman after stimulating IVF drugs have been used to produce multiple follicles (which contain eggs). These eggs are then 'frozen' using a process called vitrification, a fast form of freezing. They remain frozen until she is ready to start a family. The eggs are then defrosted and mixed with sperm in a Petri dish where the hope is that the sperm will fertilise the eggs. Once the eggs are fertilised and have developed into embryos they can be transferred into the woman's uterus where they will implant and become a fetus. This procedure is used to preserve fertility during cancer treatment and also, more recently, as a way of delaying parenting.

Embryo freezing is normally part of the standard IVF cycle. The procedure is the same as for egg freezing, except that the eggs are fertilised with the sperm before they are frozen. These embryos can be used at a later date if the first cycle of IVF fails, or used for the couple to extend their family later on after a successful pregnancy.

There is plenty of data on frozen embryos and many children have been conceived in this way. In recent years, vitrification has resulted in more embryos surviving the freezing and thawing process. Some clinics freeze embryos and do not transfer a fresh embryo, particularly in the case of older patients and in patients who suffer from OHSS (ovarian hyperstimulation syndrome). In my clinic we are advocates, under certain conditions, of delaying transfer and transferring a previously frozen embryo on a non-stimulated cycle, using acupuncture to support the endometrium and improve implantation rates.

We have much less data on egg freezing than embryo freezing; the hope is that it will one day offer women the chance to delay parenting. The data from other countries is looking promising with Spain showing 80 per cent of eggs surviving the thawing process and a 30 per cent live birth rate. The likelihood of egg freezing being successful is dependent on the age the eggs are frozen at. Freezing eggs in your late thirties may not offer you the protection that you seek.

Acupuncture during IVF

During the IVF cycle, I give acupuncture in the Stimulation phase to help pelvic blood flow and encourage the follicles to grow evenly on both sides. I advise eating plenty of good protein and Blood-nourishing foods (*see page 33*), and getting plenty of rest.

If a patient has had difficulties with egg collection in previous cycles, I may suggest acupuncture the day before to help with relaxation. Acupuncture in between egg collection and transfer is used to help with blood flow, relieve bloating and encourage receptivity. Warming foods are encouraged (*see page 30*), as is keeping warm and relaxed. I also see patients in the days after transfer to help calm the mind during the two-week wait. I have included below lots of additional tips for keeping the mind calm, and helping with the symptoms that women commonly report to me during IVF cycles, from headaches to constipation and problems sleeping.

Deep-breathing technique

Spending time each day, perhaps when you get home from work, remembering to breathe properly is deeply relaxing. I love yoga and try to do my practice two or three times a week. Observing how the breath enters and leaves the body will bring more Qi (energy) into the body and help all the body's vital functions. I like to lie on my bed with my left hand on my heart and my right on my lower belly and gently breathe between the two. I imagine the energy from my heart travelling to my uterus and back again in a continual cycle between the two centres.

Meditation

It is really important to focus on why you want a baby. It's easy to get stuck on the 'what' you want, but when you focus on the why you want a baby you really open your heart to that energy. I have seen this many times in patients who have tried for a long, long time and have lost their way a little. A simple daily meditation focusing on all the reasons why you want a baby can bring great benefits.

So many of us are control freaks, but it creates a tension within us. Sometimes the biggest shifts happen when we stop trying to control other people or circumstances around us and just accept things as they are. When we get stuck in a cycle of control we seek to control things that are beyond our control, and the more out of control we feel the more controlling we become! So kick back and try to go with the flow; you might be surprised at the gifts you find along the way.

Ways to improve our energy (Qi)

Finding ways to optimise, improve and preserve Qi (energy) is something of a national obsession in China. Qi is the building block for good health; good Qi equals long life and good fertility. Many therapies, foods and exercises are designed to help promote good QI.

Breathing fresh air

Lack of oxygen and therefore lack of Qi obtained through breath is a big problem. Many people breathe very poorly (shallowly) and the quality of air we breathe is often not ideal. Taking a stroll in country-side and being among trees and greenery is vital to our wellbeing and our Qi. If we sit slumped over a computer all day and don't get a chance to walk in nature our Qi will surely suffer. If you do have an office job and don't get outside much make sure you have some plants in your room and that you get outside at weekends.

Nourishing our emotions

When we feel well nourished emotionally everything is all right with the world; we have a lightness of heart, plenty of energy and a spring in our step. But when our needs are not met either by ourselves or through circumstance this can really begin to drain our energy. Just as we spend time working, eating, exercising and socialising, I believe it is important that we invest time into our emotional wellness. This could be through meditation or some form of therapy or simply by pursuing things that bring us joy and happiness. If you find that you are emotionally and physically fatigued you would do well to spend a little time looking inward where you may well find the source of your tiredness.

Mood boards

Mood boards are a great way to focus on what we want in our life and a visual way to bring that energy in. It's really therapeutic to collect images and scraps of fabric and words that appeal to you and put them together on a board. Then spend some time every day looking at the board and focusing on bringing that energy into your life. Designers use this tool all the time and graphic designers use mood boards to enable them to illustrate visually the direction of style that they are pursuing.

I think it is best not to think too much about it when you first start, be quite free with it. It is a creative thing to do through the IVF process to help you focus on why you are doing this. There isn't really a right or a wrong, but sometimes you might notice something quite interesting that comes out of it.

It need not be all about babies, but of course if this helps then go for it. I made a food mood board when I was starting out on this book. I put up loads of images of dishes of food or lush-looking vegetables. I noticed how natural and rural lots of my images were; I guess this is to offset my very urban lifestyle and part of something that is in my heart that I identify more with as I get older. Emma the country girl! (It's quite a small part of me but it is nice to acknowledge her every now and then.)

Observe what you place in the centre of the board – I tend to see this as a central issue, something of importance. I have quite often readjusted the central image after constructing the board as it might be something I am giving more attention than I need to. Sometimes I find when I shift that image from the central position and replace it with something else then things change.

Emotional preparation for IVF

I place such importance on the state of the mind in preparing for IVF. At a physical level, being overly stressed may create high levels of cortisol in the body, which may result in too much oestrogen. I also believe that creating a mindful state of receptiveness may be of benefit during the post-transfer two-week wait period.

Before beginning IVF, it is natural to feel anxious and have many questions about what may or may not happen. Whether you will produce embryos; will fertilisation occur; will implantation be successful. Make sure you give yourself space and time. Keep your diary quieter than normal and avoid situations that will add stress.

If you are going through IVF with a partner, use that support and be there for each other at every stage. Don't try to fit in too much around the process; take as much time as possible to take care of yourselves. Understand that everyone handles what is happening in their own way; if one of you wants to talk about it constantly but you know your partner needs to switch off every now and then, let them do just that. Be yourselves and support each other, together.

If you are going through IVF as a single person, accept the support of those closest to you to the degree that you need. Be with the people who you feel most relaxed around. Put yourself first during this time.

Be well rested and make sure that you don't have too much stress around you. Keep things as simple as you can.

How to get a good night's sleep

Things to avoid
- Eating too late.
- Serious discussions close to bedtime.
- Working late.
- Sleeping pills.
- Alcohol and smoking.

Things to do
- Go to bed early.
- Keep your bedroom as dark as possible.
- Spend some time taking a bath or doing relaxation exercises before you go to bed rather than watching TV or reading.
- Keep electrical equipment to the bare minimum in your bedroom.

Sleep

Getting a good, relaxed night's sleep is really important during IVF. Don't underestimate the rejuvenating powers of good sleep to both body and mind. Research has shown that a lack of sufficient sleep may harm your body's ability to heal and fight off illness. It will affect your levels of focus and concentration, and your moods, and will feed into your stress levels.

In Chinese medicine we interpret a lack of sleep as a factor that may deplete Qi, just like stress and overwork. And good sleep helps to build good Qi, essential throughout IVF and pregnancy.

Western research suggests that between six and seven hours of sleep is the minimum that will allow the body to experience the four essential stages of sleep, and that for adults between seven and nine hours a night is optimum.

I also place great emphasis on how we prepare for sleep – whether we wind down during the hours before sleep or go to bed still buzzing from the day. You will know how long you need personally to feel well rested and energised on waking.

Constipation

So many women complain of constipation during IVF and it can be really distressing and uncomfortable. Extra progesterone is usually the cause and this is given in order to maintain a healthy endometrium and aid the successful implantation of the embryo.

During IVF constipation is normally a result of Stagnation of energy and this responds really well to acupuncture. Abdominal self-massage is also a useful practice; use some olive oil with a couple of drops of grapefruit and orange peel essential oils.

Tea made from orange peel, fennel seeds and mint (fresh leaves) is a great remedy for constipation. Put about ten mint leaves and a teaspoon of orange peel and a teaspoon of fennel seeds into a teapot and seep for five minutes. After transfer just use orange and mint and omit the fennel seeds.

Other foods that can help with constipation include: vegetables (eat more of these and reduce refined foods), pulses, honey in warm water, prunes, raisins, rhubarb, flax seeds (soak in water overnight and add to breakfast cereal or porridge).

Headaches

Tension headaches or headaches caused by the changes in hormones are quite common during IVF. Relaxation techniques such as yoga and meditation can be helpful, as can acupuncture. Getting outside in nature or going for a swim can be a great way to move the energy and reduces tension headaches.

Certain foods have been shown to negatively affect the frequency and severity of headaches and migraine pain, including: dairy, chocolate, peanut butter, avocado, banana, citrus and onions, as well as meats with nitrates (such as bacon and hot dogs) and foods containing monosodium glutamate. Buckwheat is helpful soaked or ground and added to food or smoothies.

Four drops of lavender oil can be used diluted in a bowl of hot water and inhaled.

Bloating

The stimulation drugs can cause the energy to build up in the abdomen and many women suffer from bloating during IVF, which I regularly diagnose as either Stagnation of Qi or Dampness. This is likely to peak towards the end of the 10–14 days of stimulation and cause great discomfort.

Signs of Stagnation of Qi
- Tight abdomen or drum-like or distended abdomen.
- A desire to stretch.
- Sighing.
- Irritability.
- Mauve tongue.

Remedies for Stagnation of Qi
- Drink tangerine peel or fennel tea.
- Add fennel, tangerine, watercress and mustard cress to recipes.
- Simplify meals and avoid wheat and gluten.
- Drink warm water with a little apple cider vinegar on rising, or hot water and lemon.
- Make roasted vegetables, Carrot, Sweet Potato & Coriander Soup (*see page 149*), Sweet Chestnut Congee (*see page 207*) or a salad dressing of lemon juice, olive oil and cayenne pepper.
- Gentle exercise is good – walks will help.
- Bathe in water with a few drops of lavender oil.
- Do something creative and have fun – it helps move the Stagnation and the feelings of 'stuckness'.

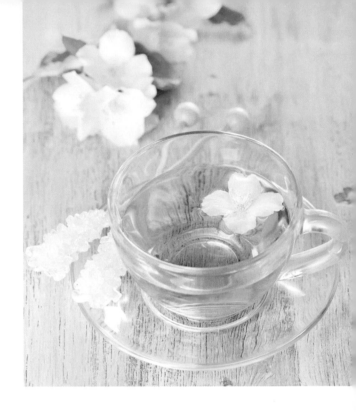

Signs of Dampness

- Watery distension.
- Being off-form.
- Damp to touch.
- Experiencing general discomfort.
- Digestive disturbance.
- Fuzzy-headed.
- Heavy feeling.
- Tiredness.
- The tongue may be coated, yellow or white.

Remedies for Dampness

- Drink barley water.
- Drink jasmine tea.

Acupuncture

Acupuncture at this time is really beneficial and often overlooked as many people focus on the before and after embryo transfer. I often have patients come in with protruding abdomens that literally deflate an inch in front of your eyes after acupuncture. It is really important to try and reduce the bloating prior to embryo transfer, as if you become pregnant the increase in hormones can cause the bloating to progress. If acupuncture is not easily accessible follow the dietary suggestions on the previous page.

Beetroot and IVF

Beetroot is rich in nitrates and a good source of iron, folate, betaine, magnesium and other anti-oxidants (particularly betacyanin). Studies have indicated that nitrate supplementation through drinking beetroot juice improves blood flow. Drinking beetroot juice could be beneficial for women undergoing IVF with thin uterine lining by increasing nutrient-rich blood flow to the uterus and ovaries.[1] Beet Kvass (*see page 213*) is a good drink to try as it has the added benefit of containing probiotics. This concurs with Chinese medicine thinking that beetroots are an excellent Blood-nourishing food.

Male Fertility and IVF

Sperm takes three months to develop in the testes and so, by the time you are at the IVF stage, the sperm will be formed and ready for fertilising the eggs collected during IVF. Sometimes ICSI is used when the sperm is unable to fertilise the egg; the sperm is injected into the egg then left to develop for three or five days. Any nutrition or lifestyle programme designed to improve the male factor needs to start at least three months prior to IVF. (S*ee pages 101–108 for a full exploration of optimising*

male fertility.) However, even improving your lifestyle at the time of IVF may help the mitochondria aspect of the sperm. So, no excuses for either of you not being healthy during the cycle itself!

What to eat during IVF

During the two-week stimulation phase we need to increase blood flow to the uterus and to the follicles. This is very much like the NOURISH stage of the menstrual cycle. Now is the time to support the body by eating Blood- and Yin-nourishing foods (*see the lists on page 48*). The menu plan below gives you an example of a good diet to follow during this period.

After the embryo transfer takes place will come the dreaded two-week wait. Now we need warmth to aid implantation – so this is like the WARM stage of the menstrual cycle. (*See page 50 for the list of warming foods.*) Cooked warm foods will warm the body and help incubate an implanting embryo.

IVF Support menu plan

DAY	BREAKFAST	LUNCH	DINNER	SUGGESTED SNACKS
1	Warm water with lemon *and* Quinoa, Chia Seed & Cardamom Porridge with Coconut, Pistachios & Raspberries (*see page 134*)	Baked Feta with Vegetable Spaghetti (*see page 202*)	Dahl with Roasted Tomatoes (*see page 154*)	Turmeric Milk (*see page 212*) Cannonball (any) (*see pages 209–210*) Beet Kvass (*see page 213*)
2	Warm water with lemon *and* scrambled eggs with Nut, Spice & Seed Mix (*see page 168*)	Kidney Bean, Quinoa & Leek Salad with Toasted Pumpkin Seeds (*see page 195*)	Chicken, Asparagus & Tarragon Soup (*see page 151*) **Vegetarian option:** Celeriac & Chestnut Soup with Chestnut & Herb Pesto (*see page 147*)	Turmeric Milk (*see page 212*) Cannonball (any) (*see pages 209–210*) Beet Kvass (*see page 213*)
3	Warm water with lemon *and* Mixed Grain Porridge with Blackberries, Hazelnuts & Flaxseeds (*see page 133*)	Roasted Bone Marrow with Shallot & Parsley Salad (*see page 182*) **Vegetarian option:** White Beans with Wilted Greens (*see page 197*)	Saffron Fish & Vegetable Stew (*see page 180*) **Vegetarian option:** Carrot, Sweet Potato & Coriander Soup (*see page 149*)	Turmeric Milk (*see page 212*) Cannonball (any) (*see pages 209–210*) Beet Kvass (*see page 213*)

DAY	BREAKFAST	LUNCH	DINNER	SUGGESTED SNACKS
4	Warm water with lemon *and a* smashed avocado and poached egg on rye bread	Butternut Squash, Chestnut & Seaweed Risotto (*see page 196*) served with a little Green Kraut (*see page 162*)	Aduki Bean, Tomato & Miso Soup (*see page 148*)	Turmeric Milk (*see page 212*) Cannonball (any) (*see pages 209–210*) Beet Kvass (*see page 213*)
5	Warm water with lemon *and* Baked Porridge with Goji Berries & Cinnamon (*see page 135*)	Caponata with Toasted Almonds (*see page 189*) served with a little Green Kraut (*see page 162*)	Avocado Soup with Crabmeat (*see page 150*) **Vegetarian option:** Avocado Soup (*see page 150*)	Turmeric Milk (*see page 212*) Cannonball (any) (*see pages 209–210*) Beet Kvass (*see page 213*)
6	Warm water with lemon *and* Sweet Chestnut Congee (*see page 207*)	Roasted Sardines with Tomato, Onion & Pomegranate (*see page 177*) served with a little Golden Kraut (*see page 161*) **Vegetarian option:** Sweet Potato & Chickpea Gnocchi (*see page 200*) with Brazil Nut & Rocket Pesto (*see page 166*)	Spiced Paneer with Wilted Greens (*see page 199*) served with brown rice	Turmeric Milk (*see page 212*) Cannonball (any) (*see pages 209–210*) Beet Kvass (*see page 213*)
7	Warm water with lemon *and* Black Sesame Porridge with Roasted Saffron Peaches (*see page 136*)	Baked Eggs with Vegetables (*see page 140*)	Beef Shin & Pumpkin Stew (*see page 181*) **Vegetarian option:** Three-bean Tagine with Almond & Lemon Couscous (*see page 192*)	Turmeric Milk (*see page 212*) Cannonball (any) (*see pages 209–210*) Beet Kvass (*see page 213*)

RECIPES

Good nutrition is my mission and good food is my passion. The recipes in this section are intended to help you to create a more healthy relationship with the food that you eat. I hope you enjoy them.

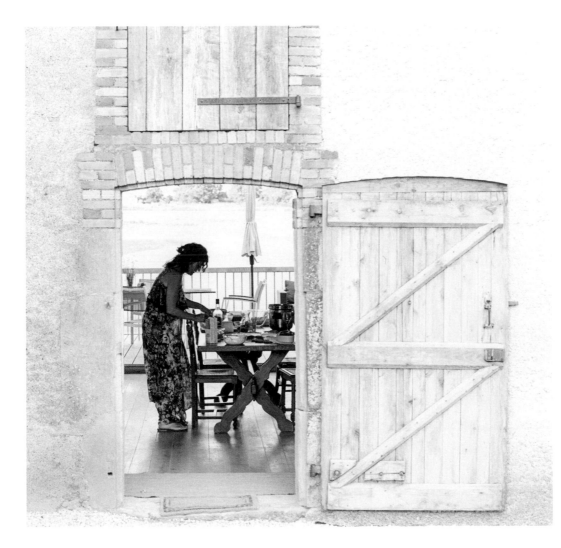

Food for optimal fertility and digestive health

Delicious food and baby making go hand in hand. Taking pleasure in what you eat and taking time to prepare nutritious meals for yourself and your loved one will not only bring you joy but will also help your body function better and create the best possible conditions for making a new life.

In this section you will find a wide variety of recipes that nutritionist Victoria Wells and I have developed with optimal fertility and digestive health in mind. All the recipes in the menu planners are on the following pages. Between them they contain all the nutrients you need for healthy eggs and sperm, as well as good general health, with none of the nasties that can do you damage.

A typical processed meal may contain ingredients from all over the world and the produce – meat, vegetables and fish – may have been transported and stored frozen for months before it is used in the end dish. Even the ingredients of a simple so-called healthy loaf of wholegrain bread may contain a cocktail of artificial additives that reduce the microbial diversity of your gut.

Our recipes encourage you to use fresh, organic produce. My preference would always be that you eat a hearty breakfast and a decent lunch and then have a lighter dinner by 7pm. I know this is not always possible, but eating the biggest meal of the day at 9pm and then going to bed shortly afterwards will wreck your digestion and cause lots of problems with absorption. So even moderating my ideal will bring health benefits.

I really want you to adapt the plans and recipes to suit your lifestyle and not become too rigid. Rigidity will cause problems in and of itself, so please do be relaxed around food. You can of course swap eggs from breakfast and eat them for lunch or supper. I often have soup for breakfast, especially a nice chicken broth. Soup is suitable at any time of day in my book! Any of these meals can be adapted and customised to make them more suitable to your condition. Black sesame seeds sprinkled on vegetables will increase the Blood-nourishing quality of the food. Spices added will bring warmth, adding fermented foods helps move Stagnation, and so on. There are so many little ways you can tweak the recipes to make them more bespoke to you. Think of it like alchemy; the sum of the parts is greater than the individual components.

Equally, don't become a slave to the ingredients. If you go to the market and you see an ingredient that looks delicious, go for it. You will probably invent something amazing inspired by the book and what your eyes are drawn to. Remember that eating starts with the senses, so follow them.

How to eat well

For nutritious eating, the plate should be mainly plant-based with a little high-quality meat included in your weekly diet. Eat good dairy including traditional cheeses, yoghurts and kefir. Cook mainly with second-pressed olive oil, use cold-pressed oils for adding to food after cooking and eat a wide variety of nuts, vegetables and pulses to provide lots of healthy fibre. Limit sugar intake from juices and other drinks and have other sweet foods, such as dark chocolate and cakes, as an occasional treat.

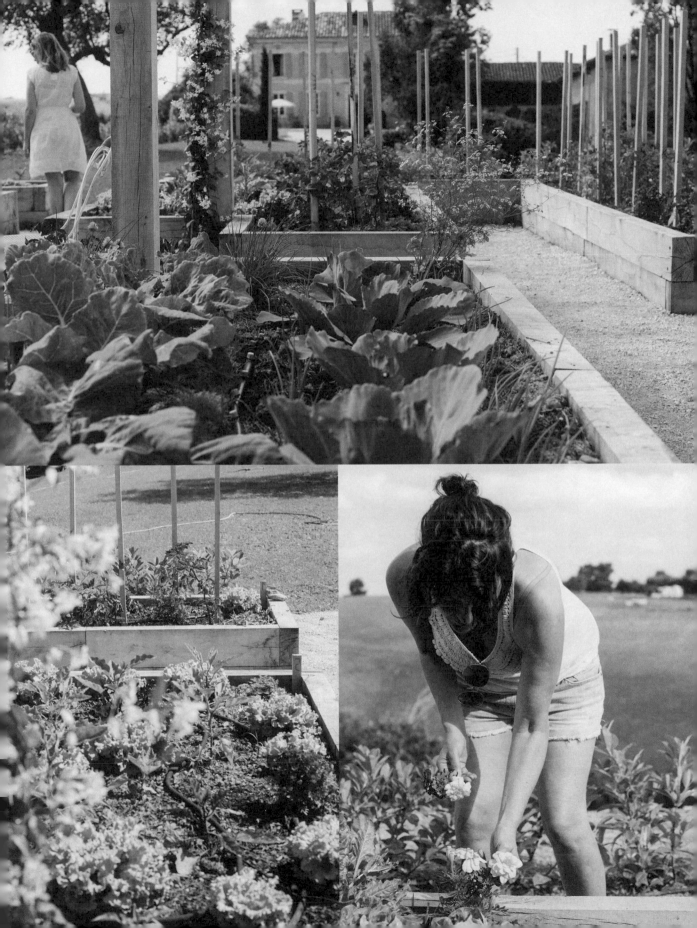

Eating five to eight servings of fruit and vegetables daily with a range of nuts and seeds will ensure you absorb adequate antioxidant nutrients. Antioxidants reduce levels of free radicals and modulate the body's inflammatory response. As a general rule, try to make your plate colourful with a variety of seasonal fruits and vegetables especially red, black and blue types of berries, tomatoes, citrus fruits and dark green leafy vegetables. Also ensure you eat cruciferous vegetables including pak choi, broccoli, cauliflower, Brussels sprouts, cabbage and kale. Do eat organic when you can. Organic fruits and vegetables can contain as much as 70 per cent more antioxidants than non-organic. A study published in 2016 by the *British Journal of Nutrition* found that organic fruits and vegetables can contain as much as 70 per cent more antioxidants than non-organic. The authors of the study estimated a switch to organic could boost antioxidant consumption by between 20 and 40 per cent.

Probiotics and prebiotics consumed daily will nourish and nurture your microbial garden. Good sources include kefir, sauerkraut and prebiotic- and polyphenol-rich plant foods. Ensure your diet includes a wide variety of vegetables, darkly coloured berries, nuts (particularly chestnut and hazelnut), seeds and fresh herbs and spices. Add these liberally to cooking, particularly cloves, star anise and oregano. Diversity is key. And perhaps most important of all for a healthy gut – try the recipes for fermenting food at home, such as Sauerkraut and Beet Kvass. Fermenting preserves seasonal vegetables and also increases their nutrient profile. Fermented foods restore your gut to health, help manage weight loss and can even improve your mood and feelings of wellbeing. No less than 70 per

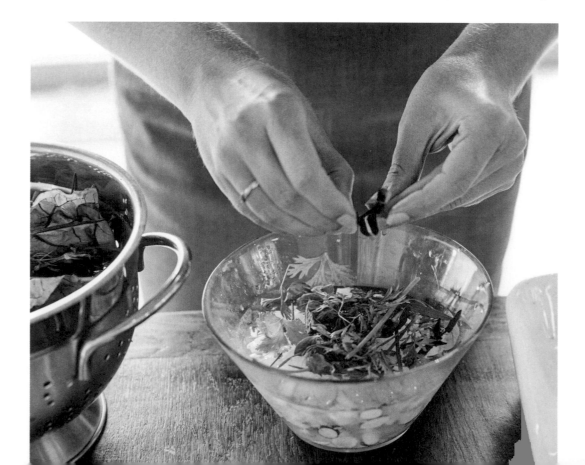

cent of the serotonin in your body is produced in your gut! Food fermented at home has a wider microbial diversity than shop-bought versions.

Weekly food preparation need not be a chore – it can be a ritual. Instead of randomly selecting meals on the hoof, start to get into the habit of planning them so they flow from one to another. Roast a chicken on Sunday and then use the bones and leftover meat for a chicken noodle soup on Monday night. Think ahead and soak wholegrains overnight to increase their digestibility and reduce cooking time the next day. Prepare overnight oats for a ready-made (and transportable) breakfast the next morning. Set aside a little time to bulk sauté onions and leeks. If you double up recipes and freeze the rest you can cook half as often!

Above all, savour your meals. Taking the time to fully plan, prepare and digest will reap enormous benefits for you both now and in future life.

The most important meal of the day

Starting the day with breakfast is associated with healthy eating for the rest of the day. Breakfast boosts energy levels and helps you manage hunger and stabilise blood sugar. Boxed breakfast cereals are not the best option, however; many breakfast cereals are said to contain less nutrition than the boxes they come in! They certainly can be laden with sugar and the so-called healthier varieties often have superfood gimmicky claims on the packet to distract us from how nutrient poor they really are. While many boxed cereals are enriched with nutrients, the bioavailability of these is poor – in other words, the nutrients are not optimally absorbed by our bodies.

Eggs

Eggs are powerhouses of key nutrients including high quality protein, unsaturated fatty acids, vitamin D, vitamin B12, vitamin A, selenium and choline. The nutrients are concentrated in the egg yolk and long-standing notions that the egg yolk was bad news for heart health have been rethought. Eggs are good poached, fried, boiled, scrambled and baked, and eaten throughout the day, not only at breakfast.

I often add vegetables to my breakfast. It helps you increase your intake and adds a burst of flavour that deserves a prominent place on your breakfast plate. Think wilted greens, stir-fried kale, sliced avocado, steamed asparagus, roasted tomatoes and sautéed mushrooms.

Porridge

I eat porridge a couple of times a week in the Winter. My favourite way to eat it is with butter and honey. Porridge is a good way to introduce a wider range of wholegrains into your diet. Porridge can be defined as a grain cooked in water or milk. The grains used differ around the world and you can use cracked, rolled or ground grains. Add mixed seeds, nuts, poached spiced fruits, fresh seasonal berries or even pumpkin or carrot. These porridges are a long way from plain unappetising gruel!

Foods to help balance and nourish your body

Effect	Foods
Cooling	Apples, aubergines, bitter salad leaves, cottage cheese, crab, cress, cucumbers, grapefruit, lemons, lettuce, milk (cow's or soya), mung bean soup, mussels, pears, pork, raw tomatoes, spinach, tofu, yoghurt.
Damp-resolving	Aduki beans, alfalfa sprouts (avoid all sprouts when pregnant), asparagus, barley, basil, buckwheat, caraway, cardamom, celery, coriander, corn, endives, horseradish, lemons, parsley.
Warming	Almonds, beetroot, carrots, cayenne pepper, chicken, chocolate, cinnamon, cloves, cooked tomatoes, figs, garlic, ginger, lamb, peaches, peppers, mustard, nutmeg, pumpkins, radishes, sesame seeds, squash.
Blood-nourishing	Aduki beans, apricots, beef, beetroot, bone broth, bone marrow, cherries, dandelion, dates, eggs, figs, grapes, kale, kidney beans, leafy greens, mussels, nettles, octopus, oysters, parsley, sardines, seaweed, squid, sweet rice, tempeh, watercress.
Blood-moving	Aubergines, chestnuts, chilli, chives, crab, eggs, kohlrabi, leeks, liver, mustard leaves, onions, peaches, radishes, saffron, spring onions, sticky rice, turmeric, vinegar.
Stimulating	Almonds, caraway, cardamom, carrots, cayenne pepper, chicken, coconut, dates, eggs, fennel seeds, figs, grapes, lentils, millet, molasses, oats, quinoa, rice, sage, sardines, shiitake mushrooms, star anise, squash, tangerine peel.
Kidney-nourishing	Alfalfa, asparagus, chestnuts, eggs, kidney beans, nettles, oats, quinoa, string beans, walnuts.
Jing-nourishing	Almonds, artichokes, bone broth, bone marrow, chicken, clams, eggs, full-fat organic milk, kidneys, liver, mackerel, mussels, oysters, pistachio nuts, seaweed, scallops, sesame seeds, walnuts.
Qi-nourishing	Almonds, aromatic seeds (caraway, cardamom, coriander, fennel), carrots, cherries, chickpeas, coconut, eggs, lentils, liquorice, mackerel, milk, millet, molasses, oats, potatoes, quinoa, rice, sage, sardines, sweet potatoes, shiitake mushrooms, squash, tofu, trout, venison, yam.
Yin-nourishing	Apples, asparagus, avocados, cheese, clams, crab, duck, eggs, green beans, honey, lemons, malt, mangoes, milk, nettles, oysters, pears, pineapple, pomegranates, pork, seaweed, sesame seeds, spelt, spinach, tomatoes, watermelons, wheat, yam.

The benefits of cinnamon

Cinnamon not only adds a subtle sweet flavour to porridge, it may help improve blood glucose levels and increase insulin sensitivity. There is evidence that cinnamon slows the rate at which the stomach empties after meals.

I hope you will try a wide variety of grains but you can substitute the grains in the recipes on pages 130–134 for simple rolled-oats if necessary. The general rule of thumb when making porridge is a 2:1 ratio. That's two parts liquid to one part grain. If the porridge looks too thick add a little water.

Soaking grains

Phytic acid is present in grains (legumes and raw nuts) and therefore it is important to soak these foods to break down phytic acid in order to aid digestion. Phytic acid binds to minerals as the foods are being digested and this limits absorption. Soaking also increases the digestibility of grains and helps reduce bloating.

How to soak grains

- Place the grains in a large bowl. Pour over plenty of filtered water and cover the bowl with a plate or cloth.
- All grains need soaking for 12 hours except millet, brown rice and buckwheat, which have less phytic acid and only require seven hours.
- Leave for the allotted time and then drain and gently rinse
- Soaked grains often need less cooking time than non-soaked grains

Bone broth

I'm a believer in nose to tail eating philosophy. Part of the natural rhythm of cooking starts with not wasting a thing. For carnivores this includes offal in all its glory and never ever wasting the bones.

Broth is nourishing and soothing to the digestion. It has a long reputation as a traditional healing food and it may help with inflammation and digestive problems. Made at home, it is nutrient-dense, providing amino acids, minerals and the proteins collagen and cartilage. You can make it in large quantities to be used in different ways: as a base for soups and other dishes and as a drink by itself. When you make a batch of broth for stock (*see page 142*), it's a good idea to freeze some in ice-cube trays to add to your cooking to enrich dishes like stews and wholegrains.

Bone Broth Drink

Bone broth is warming and satisfying. Try it as a mid-morning, afternoon or evening drink. To make the a bone broth drink, pour 350 ml (12 fl oz) Chicken Broth (see *page 142*) into a small pan and cook over low heat for 5 minutes until heated through. Pour the broth into a mug, stir in either ¼ teaspoon of grated fresh root ginger, ¼ teaspoon of grated turmeric root or a pinch of chilli flakes and let infuse for 2 minutes before drinking.

A note on ingredients

- I have used whole milk or kefir in the breakfast recipes. If you cannot tolerate milk use unsweetened almond milk or coconut milk.
- Standard level spoon measurements are used in all recipes:

  1 tablespoon = one 15 ml spoon

  1 teaspoon = one 5 ml spoon.
- Both imperial and metric measurements have been given in all recipes. Use one set of measurements only and not a mixture of both.
- Eggs should be medium unless otherwise stated. The Department of Health advises that eggs should not be consumed raw.
- Always check the labels of preprepared ingredients to make sure they do not contain ingredients that are not suitable if you are following a vegetarian, vegan, gluten-free or low-carb diet. For vegetarian recipes, check cheese labels to ensure they are suitable for vegetarians and use vegetarian Parmesan-style cheese instead of traditional Parmesan, which is made with animal rennet.

Breakfasts

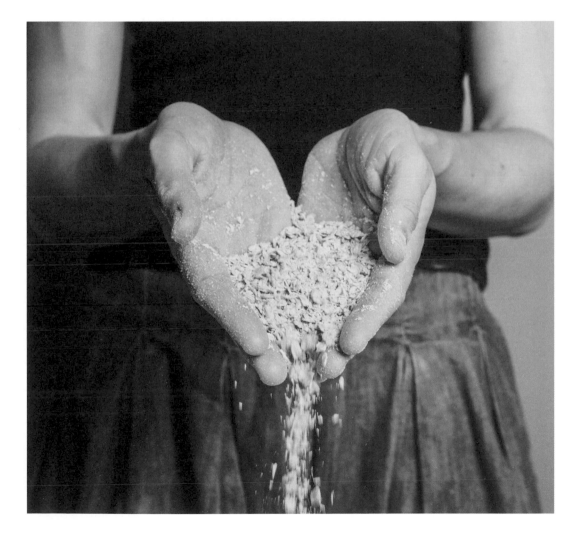

AMARANTH, SPICED PEAR & PUMPKIN SEED PORRIDGE

Serves 2

100 g (3½ oz) amaranth, soaked
  overnight in filtered water
  (*see page 127*) and drained
475 ml (16 fl oz) milk (use
  whichever type of milk you
  prefer)
2 pears, peeled, cored, and diced
2 tsp ground cinnamon
¼ tsp ground nutmeg
¼ tsp vanilla extract
1 tbsp freshly squeezed orange
  juice

To serve
2 tbsp honey
2 tbsp pumpkin seeds

Amaranth is a gluten-free grain. It is actually a tiny seed but is cultivated as a grain.

Put the amaranth into a heavy-based pan, pour over the milk and bring to the boil, then reduce the heat, cover with a lid and simmer for 25 minutes, checking occasionally and adding a little filtered water if the porridge is too dry. Remove from the heat and let stand for 5 minutes.

Meanwhile, put the pear, cinnamon, nutmeg, vanilla extract and orange juice into a small pan and cook over low heat for 10–12 minutes until softened.

Mix the stewed pear into the porridge. Divide the porridge between 2 bowls, drizzle with the honey, sprinkle over the pumpkin seeds and serve immediately.

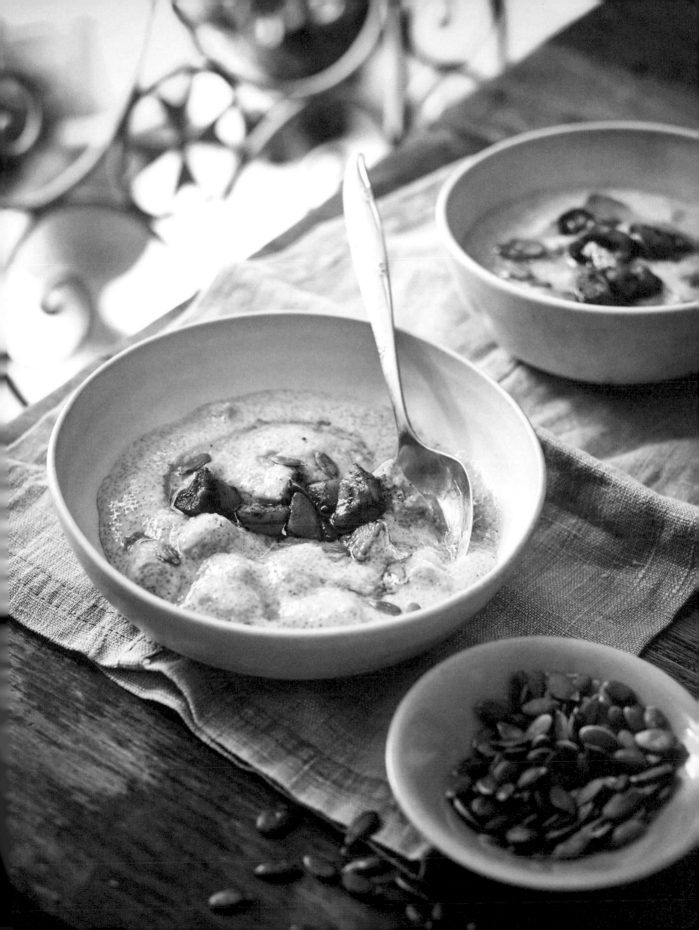

RECIPES

SPICED PUMPKIN & QUINOA PORRIDGE

Serves 2

100 g (3½ oz) quinoa, rinsed
450 ml (¾ pint) milk (use whichever
   type of milk you prefer)
50 ml (2 fl oz) filtered water
125 g (4 oz) pumpkin purée
2 tsp black sesame seeds
1 tsp ground cinnamon
¼ tsp ground ginger

To serve

2 tbsp chopped pecan nuts
a little honey (optional)

Put the quinoa into a bowl with the milk, cover with
a plate or tea towel and let soak overnight.

The next day, transfer the soaked quinoa and milk to
a heavy-based pan, add the filtered water and bring to
the boil. Add the pumpkin purée, sesame seeds, cinnamon
and ginger, reduce the heat and simmer for 15–20 minutes,
stirring frequently, until the porridge is your desired
consistency, adding a little extra water if the porridge
becomes too thick. Remove from the heat, cover with a lid
and let stand for 5 minutes.

To serve, divide the porridge between 2 bowls, sprinkle over
the pecan nuts and drizzle with a little honey, if using.

This warming and nourishing porridge tastes great and is really
beneficial to the digestive system. The quinoa is a complete source
of protein and the pumpkin is rich in beta-carotene for sperm quality
and count.

MIXED GRAIN PORRIDGE WITH BLACKBERRIES, HAZELNUTS & FLAXSEEDS

Serves 2

100 g (3½ oz) mixed grains (try buckwheat, porridge oats and quinoa), soaked overnight in filtered water (*see page 127*) and drained

475 ml (16 fl oz) milk (use whichever type of milk you prefer)

To serve

3 tbsp blackberries
2 tbsp chopped hazelnuts
1 heaped tbsp flaxseeds
a little honey (optional)

Using a mixture of grains in your porridge adds texture and provides a wider variety of nutrients and flavours.

Put the grains into a heavy-based pan, pour over the milk and bring to the boil, then reduce the heat and simmer for 15–20 minutes, stirring frequently, until the porridge is your desired consistency. Add little filtered water if the porridge becomes too thick.

To serve, divide the porridge between 2 bowls, sprinkle over the blackberries, hazelnuts and flaxseeds and drizzle with a little honey, if using.

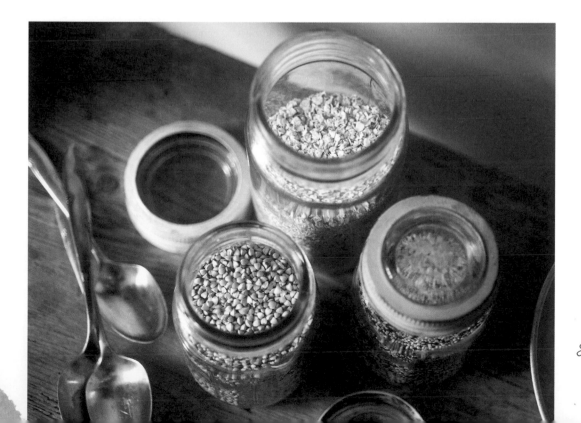

QUINOA, CHIA SEED & CARDAMOM PORRIDGE WITH COCONUT, PISTACHIOS & RASPBERRIES

Serves 2

100 g (3½ oz) quinoa, rinsed
2 tsp chia seeds
300 ml (½ pint) milk (use whichever type of milk you prefer)
300 ml coconut milk
¼ tsp ground cardamom
½ tsp ground cinnamon

To serve

1 tbsp crushed roasted pistachios
2 tbsp raspberries
1 tbsp coconut chips
1 banana, sliced
a little maple syrup

Chia seeds are packed with nutrients including protein, fibre and omega-3s. They are useful in cooking as the seeds form a gel when mixed with liquid and can be used as a thickener.

Put the quinoa and chia seeds into a bowl with the milk, cover with a plate or tea towel and let soak overnight.

The next day, transfer the soaked quinoa and chia seeds and the milk to a heavy-based pan, add the coconut milk and cardamom and bring to the boil, then reduce the heat and simmer for 15–20 minutes, stirring continuously, until the porridge is your desired consistency. Add a little filtered water if the porridge becomes too dry. Remove from the heat, cover with a lid and let stand for 5 minutes.

To serve, divide the porridge between 2 bowls, sprinkle over the pistachios, raspberries, coconut, and banana and drizzle with a little maple syrup.

BAKED PORRIDGE WITH GOJI BERRIES & CINNAMON

Serves 2

120 g (4 oz) oatmeal

2 tbsp goji berries

30 g (1¼ oz) pumpkin seeds or mixed seeds

2 tsp black sesame seeds

1 tsp ground cinnamon

300 ml (½ pint) milk (use whichever type of milk you prefer) or filtered water

butter, for greasing

2 tbsp grated orange zest

To serve

kefir

a little honey

Put the oatmeal, goji berries, pumpkin or mixed seeds, sesame seeds and cinnamon into a bowl with the milk or water, cover with a plate or tea towel and let soak overnight.

The next day, preheat the oven to 190°C/375°C/Gas Mark 5. Generously grease an ovenproof dish with butter.

Transfer the oatmeal mixture to the prepared dish, add the orange zest and add a little hot water, if necessary, to loosen the mixture. Bake in the oven for 15 minutes, or until the porridge is your desired consistency. If the porridge is too thick, add a little more hot milk or water and return to the oven for 10 minutes.

To serve, divide the porridge between 2 bowls, pour over a little kefir to loosen the porridge and then drizzle with a little honey.

BLACK SESAME PORRIDGE WITH ROASTED SAFFRON PEACHES

Serves 2

90 g (3¼ oz) white basmati rice
30 g (1¼ oz) black sesame seeds
pinch of sea salt

For the roasted saffron peaches
2 slightly ripe but firm peaches,
    halved and pitted
pinch of saffron threads
½ tsp vanilla extract
2 tbsp honey
juice of 1 lemon

To serve
a little honey
25 g (1 oz) pistachios, toasted and
    chopped

Wash the rice under cold running tap until the water runs clear. Put the rice into a bowl with the water, cover with a plate or tea towel and let soak overnight.

The next day, rinse the rice under cold running water and drain well.

Heat a dry frying pan, add the sesame seeds and toast for a couple of minutes until they are fragrant. Transfer to a spice or coffee grinder and process to a coarse powder. Set aside.

Put the drained rice into the spice or coffee grinder and process to a coarse powder.

Put the rice powder into a heavy-based pan, add 475 ml (16 fl oz) water and bring to the boil, stirring continuously. Reduce the heat and cook over low heat for 10 minutes, stirring all the time and adding a little extra water if becomes too dry. Stir in the sesame seed powder and salt and cook until heated through.

Meanwhile, preheat the oven to 200°C/400°C/Gas Mark 6. Place the peaches, cut-side up, on a small baking sheet. Whisk together the saffron, vanilla extract, honey and lemon juice in a small bowl and spoon the mixture over the peach halves. Roast in the oven for 10–15 minutes until the peaches are bubbling and easily pierced with a butter knife.

To serve, divide the peaches and their juices between 2 bowls, spoon over the black sesame porridge, drizzle with a little honey and sprinkle over the toasted pistachios.

VARIATIONS

You can top this porridge with mixed seeds, pumpkin seeds or toasted pine nuts and replace the roasted saffron peaches with any poached seasonal fruit.

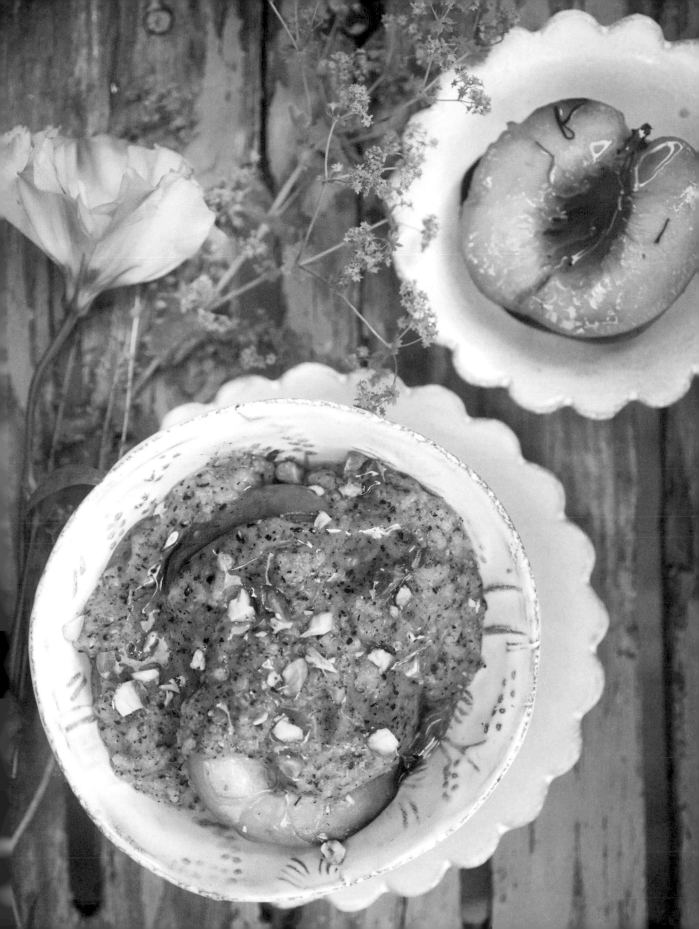

SIMPLE OVERNIGHT OATS

Serves 1

3 tbsp porridge oats
about 150 ml (¼ pint) kefir
1 tsp chia seeds

To serve
your chosen flavourings (*see box*)
a little honey

Put the oats and chia seeds into a bowl and pour over just enough kefir to cover them. Cover with a plate or tea towel and let soak overnight.

The next day, stir in your chosen flavourings and a little honey and serve. Alternatively, if you prefer to eat the overnight oats warm, transfer the oats to a pan, add a little extra kefir or some milk or water, and cook over low heat until heated through (you need to heat the oats gently in order not to destroy the gut-friendly microbes), then stir in your chosen flavourings and serve.

'CARROT CAKE' OVERNIGHT OATS

Make the simple overnight oats as above. The next day, heat 1 teaspoon coconut oil in a small frying pan, add the 1 small grated carrot and cook over medium heat for a couple of minutes until tender. Add the carrots to the overnight oat mixture, stir in a few raisins, if liked, ¼ teaspoon of ground cinnamon, ¼ teaspoon of ground cardamom, ¼ teaspoon of vanilla extract, 5 chopped walnuts and ½ tablespoon of honey.

OVERNIGHT OAT FLAVOURINGS

Natural yoghurt, fruit, nuts, seeds and spices are all great additions to overnight oats, and they can be combined in so many different ways. Here are some of my favourite flavourings:

Natural yoghurt + grated apple + chopped pear + seasonal berries + mixed seeds

Chopped pear + ground cinnamon + vanilla extract + chopped almonds

Chopped figs + chopped apple + ground cinnamon + ground ginger + chopped brazil nuts

Seasonal berries: blackberries, blueberries, raspberries, strawberries

Mixed seeds + grated apple + honey

Blackberries + chopped hazelnuts + honey

CHESTNUT COMPOTE

Makes 1 x 500-ml (17-fl oz) jar

150 g (5 oz) dried pitted apricots,
roughly chopped into thirds

150 g (5 oz) dried pitted dates,
roughly chopped into thirds

150 g (5 oz) vacuum-packed
chestnuts, halved

2 tsp rosewater

1 cinnamon stick

4 cardamom pods, crushed

The morning is the best time for sweet flavours. This compote is sweet, warming and a good tonic for the stomach. I love to serve this on yoghurt, as the spices set off the Cold energy of the yoghurt, or with porridge for the perfect winter-warmer breakfast.

Put all the ingredients into a pan with 125 ml (4 fl oz) warm water. Cook over low heat, stirring occasionally to help the fruit break down, for 30–45 minutes until it is the consistency of compote.

Transfer to sterilised jars (see below) and seal immediately. The compote can be stored for up to 2 months in the fridge.

HOW TO STERILISE JARS

To sterilise glass jars, wash them and their lids in very hot, soapy water. Place the jars and lids upside down on a roasting tin while still wet and allow them to air-dry, then place the roasting tin in an oven preheated to 140˚C/275˚C/Gas Mark 1 for 20 minutes. Remove from the oven and let cool for 10 minutes before filling the jars. Alternatively, wash the jars and lids on the hottest cycle in your dishwasher.

BAKED EGGS WITH VEGETABLES

Serves 2

1 small fennel bulb, finely sliced
½ leek, finely sliced
1 small courgette, diced
10 cherry tomatoes
2 tbsp olive oil
80 g (3 oz) spinach leaves
1 garlic clove, crushed (optional)
2 large eggs
1 tsp sumac

Preheat the oven to 200°C/400°F/Gas Mark 6.

Put the fennel, leek, courgette and tomatoes into a large ovenproof dish, drizzle over 1½ tablespoons of the oil and toss to coat. Roast in the oven for 20 minutes

Stir the spinach and garlic, if using, into the roasted vegetables and drizzle over the remaining oil. Using the back of a spoon, make two hollows among the vegetables and then crack an egg into each hollow. Sprinkle the sumac over the eggs. Return the dish to the oven for about 5 minutes until the eggs are just set. Serve immediately.

Eggs are wonderful – they are an incredibly versatile ingredient and so simple to prepare. Whenever I am ever stuck for something easy to cook I reach for the eggs.

Soups

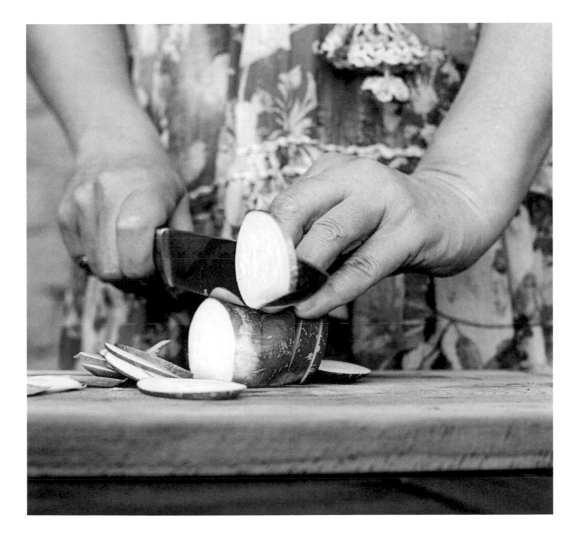

CHICKEN BROTH

Makes about 1.5 litres (2½ pints)

1 chicken carcase, weighing about
   1 kg (2 lb), plus any extra legs,
   wings or giblets if you can get
   them
2 celery sticks, including the leaves
2 brown onions, halved with the
   skins left on
2 bay leaves
3 cloves
1 slice peeled fresh root ginger
2 sprigs thyme
10 black peppercorns
1 tbsp cider vinegar

CHICKEN BROTH FLAVOURED WITH DARKENED GINGER

Heat a dry frying pan, then add ¼ teaspoon of grated fresh root ginger and cook over low heat until it changes colour but does not char. Meanwhile, pour 350 ml (12 fl oz) broth into a pan and cook over low heat for 5 minutes. Pour the broth into a mug, stir in the darkened ginger and let infuse for 2 minutes before drinking.

You can usually obtain chicken carcases from a good butcher. Other places to try are farmers' markets and vegetable delivery box companies. I don't add carrots or other root vegetables to this broth as they absorb the flavour of the meat and release little of their own flavour. Leaving out the root vegetables also results in a clearer broth. Adding a little vinegar helps extract the goodness from the bones.

If you are using a leftover roast chicken, pull off any spare meat first and set it aside to use in another dish. Reserve any juices left in the roasting pan.

Push down on the carcase until you hear the bones crack and then put them into a large stock pot or pan. Add the remaining ingredients, the roasting juices, if using, and enough cold water (about 2 litres/3½ pints) just to cover the bones – I prefer to use filtered water. Bring almost to the boil, then reduce the heat and simmer, uncovered, for 8–12 hours. Skim any froth from the surface occasionally. Let cool and then strain the broth through a fine sieve into a bowl.

The broth can be kept in the fridge for up to 5 days. Alternatively, pour the broth into ice-cube trays and freeze until ready to use.

DANG GUI CHICKEN SOUP

Serves 4–6

1 small chicken, weighing about
   1.25 kg (2½ lb)
10 g (½ oz) huang qi (astragalus
   root)
8 g (¼ oz) dang gui (angelica root)
a few slices fresh root ginger
300 ml (½ pint) black glutinous rice
   wine, such as Shaoxing rice wine
   (optional)

This soup is made using huang qi and dang gui roots, which can found in Asian stores or bought online. It is not recommended to use dang gui root if you are taking the medication Warfarin.

Bring a large pan of water to the boil. Add the chicken and cook for 5 minutes, then drain and rinse well.

Rinse the huang qi and dang gui under cold running water and then place them in a muslin bag with the ginger. Tie up the bag.

Put the chicken into a large pan, add the bag of herbs, the rice wine, if using, and enough water to cover the chicken and herbs. Cook over low heat for 6–8 hours.

Remove and discard the bag of herbs. Remove the chicken to a board and set aside until cool enough to handle. Pull the chicken meat from the bones and discard the bones and skin. Shred the meat and then return it to the broth in the pan and cook over low heat until heated through.

BEETROOT SOUP

Serves 2

1 tbsp coconut oil

1 small red onion, finely chopped

4 raw beetroot, peeled and cut into
  1-cm (½-inch) cubes (coarsely
  chop the stalks if available)

1 waxy potato, peeled and cut into
  1-cm (½-inch) cubes

1 tsp fennel seeds

1 garlic clove, crushed

500 ml (17 fl oz) Chicken Broth (*see
  page 142*) or vegetable broth

sea salt and freshly ground black
  pepper

To garnish (warm soup)

natural yoghurt, soured cream or
  crème fraîche, to serve

½ tsp freshly grated horseradish
  (optional)

1 tbsp finely chopped chives

To garnish (chilled soup)

ice cubes

sliced spring onions

sliced radishes

fresh coriander leaves

Heat the coconut oil in a large, heavy-based pan and gently sauté the onion over low heat for 5 minutes. Add the beetroot, potato, fennel seeds and garlic and stir well, then pour over the broth and bring to the boil. Reduce the heat and simmer for 15–20 minutes until the vegetables are soft. Let cool for a few minutes, then transfer the soup to a food processor and blend until smooth. Return the soup to the pan and reheat gently. Season to taste with salt and pepper.

The soup can be served either warm or chilled. If serving warm, ladle the soup into bowls, add a dollop of yoghurt, soured cream or crème fraîche to each bowl and sprinkle over the horseradish, if using, and chives. If serving cold, ladle the soup into bowls, add an ice cube or two and garnish with some sliced spring onions and radishes and a few fresh coriander leaves.

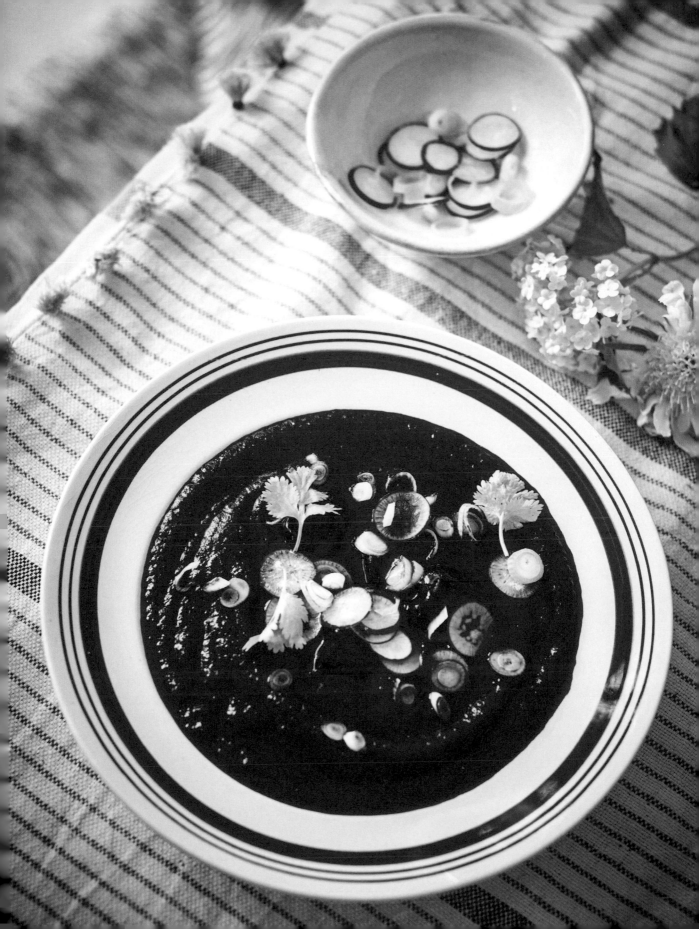

OYSTER, LEEK & SWEET POTATO SOUP WITH JAPANESE 7-SPICE POWDER

Serves 2

2 tbsp butter

2 leeks, finely sliced

1 sweet potato, peeled and diced

2.5-cm (1-inch) piece fresh ginger root, peeled and grated

2 garlic cloves, sliced

700 ml (24 fl oz) Chicken Broth (*see page 142*)

6 rock oysters

sea salt and freshly ground black pepper

For the Japanese 7-spice powder

1 tbsp black sesame seeds, toasted

1 tbsp white sesame seeds, toasted

1 ½ tbsp dried tangerine peel

2 tsp dried seaweed flakes

1 tsp poppy seeds, toasted

2 tsp Szechuan peppercorns, toasted

½ tsp ground ginger

This soup is made with our version of the Japanese 7-spice powder 'Shichimi Togarashi'. Store any leftover spice powder in an airtight container and use it to flavour meat, fish and rice dishes or add an aromatic fragrance to soups.

First make the Japanese 7-spice powder. Put all the ingredients into a spice grinder and process to a fine powder. Alternatively, you can grind the spices by hand using a pestle and mortar if you prefer a coarser texture.

Melt the butter in a large, heavy-based pan. Add the leeks, sweet potato and ginger and cook over low heat until the leeks are soft and translucent. Add the garlic and cook for an additional 2 minutes. Pour over the broth, bring to a gentle rolling boil and cook for about 10 minutes until the sweet potato is cooked. Let cool for a few minutes.

Shuck the oysters over a bowl to catch the oyster liquor. Set aside the oysters and strain the oyster liquor into a clean bowl.

Transfer the soup to a food processor and blend until smooth. Return the soup to the pan, stir in the oyster liquor and reheat gently. Season to taste with salt and pepper.

Place 3 oysters in each soup bowl and then ladle over the soup. Garnish the soup with a liberal sprinkling of Japanese 7-spice powder.

CELERIAC & CHESTNUT SOUP WITH CHESTNUT & HERB PESTO

Serves 2

1 tbsp olive oil

1 celery stick, finely chopped

1 carrot, finely chopped

1 leek, finely sliced

½ celeriac, peeled and diced

1 garlic clove, finely chopped

2 bay leaves

700 ml (24 fl oz) Chicken Broth (*see page 142*) or vegetable broth

100 g (3½ oz) vacuum-packed chestnuts

60 ml (2½ fl oz) crème fraîche

2 tbsp Chestnut & Herb Pesto (*see page 167*), to garnish

Heat the oil in a large, heavy-based pan. Add the celery, carrot and leek and sauté over low heat for 15 minutes. Add the celeriac, garlic and bay leaves and cook for 2 minutes, then pour over the broth and bring to the boil. Cover with a lid, reduce the heat and simmer for 20 minutes. Add the chestnuts and cook for 5 more minutes. Let cool for a few minutes, then transfer the soup to a food processor and blend until smooth. Return the soup to the pan, stir in the crème fraîche and reheat gently.

Ladle the soup into bowls and add a dollop of pesto on top.

This is my go-to recipe when I crave soup on an autumn evening. Chestnuts tonify the stomach energy and help create good digestion.

ADUKI BEAN, TOMATO & MISO SOUP

Serves 2

200 g (7 oz) aduki beans
150 g (5 oz) butternut squash, cut
    into 2.5-cm (1-inch) chunks
2 tbsp olive oil
1 small red onion, finely diced
1 garlic clove, crushed
1 tsp tamari soy sauce
1 tsp peeled and grated fresh root
    ginger
1 tsp miso paste
200 ml (7 fl oz) passata
500 ml (17 fl oz) Chicken Broth (*see
    page 142*) or vegetable broth

To garnish

1 handful fresh coriander leaves,
    chopped
2 tbsp natural yoghurt

You can make this soup with either aduki beans or black beans. Aduki beans tend to be more Damp-draining but both are sweet and tonifying for the digestion.

Soak the beans in a bowl of cold water overnight.

The next day, rinse and drain the beans. Put the beans into a large pan and cover with water (using 3 parts water to 1 part beans). Bring to the boil, then reduce the heat and simmer for 45 minutes–1 hour until the beans are tender. Drain and set aside.

Meanwhile, preheat the oven to 180°C/350°F/Gas Mark 4. Place the butternut squash in a large roasting tin, drizzle over 1 tablespoon of oil and toss to coat. Roast in the oven for 30 minutes, or until soft.

Heat the remaining oil in a large, heavy-based pan. Add the onion and garlic and cook over low heat for 15 minutes until soft and translucent. Add the roasted butternut squash, soy sauce, ginger, miso paste, passata and broth and bring to the boil, then reduce the heat and simmer for 5 minutes. Let cool for a few minutes, then transfer the soup to a food processor and blend until smooth. Return the soup to the pan and reheat gently.

Ladle the soup into bowls, add a dollop of yoghurt on top and sprinkle over the coriander.

CARROT, SWEET POTATO & CORIANDER SOUP

Serves 2–3

2 tsp coriander seeds
25 g (1 oz) butter or ghee
400 g (13 oz) carrots, chopped
1 sweet potato, peeled and
    chopped
1 small garlic clove, crushed
700 ml (24 fl oz) Chicken Broth (*see
    page 142*) or vegetable broth
25 g (1 oz) chopped fresh coriander
sea salt and freshly ground black
    pepper

Toast the coriander seeds in a dry frying pan for 1–2 minutes until they are fragrant. Use a mortar and pestle to coarsely crush the seeds.

Heat the butter or ghee in a large pan. Add the carrots, sweet potato, garlic and three-quarters of the crushed coriander seeds, cover with a lid and cook gently for 15 minutes. Pour over the broth and bring to the boil, then reduce the heat and simmer for 15–20 minutes until the vegetables are tender. Let cool for a few minutes, then transfer the soup to a food processor and blend until smooth. Return the soup to the pan, stir in the fresh coriander and reheat gently. Season to taste with salt and pepper.

Ladle the soup into bowls and sprinkle over the remaining crushed coriander seeds.

AVOCADO SOUP

Serves 2

1 tbsp coconut oil
1 small red onion, chopped
1 celery stick, sliced
1 small garlic clove, crushed
1 very large or 2 small ripe
   avocados
juice of 1 lime
400 ml (14 fl oz) Chicken Broth (*see
   page 142*) or vegetable broth
4 tbsp natural yoghurt
¼ tsp paprika
sea salt and freshly ground black
   pepper
1 handful fresh coriander leaves,
   chopped, to garnish

AVOCADO SOUP
WITH CRABMEAT
Make the soup as above and
ladle into bowls. Place half
the remaining avocado in the
centre of each bowl of soup,
then top with a mound of
white crab meat and garnish
with the coriander.

Avocados provide carotenoids which are associated with higher sperm motility (according to a 2013 study that measured semen quality in relation to antioxidant intake in a healthy male population). The greatest concentration of carotenoids is found in the dark green flesh underneath the avocado skin.

Heat the coconut oil in a heavy-based pan and sauté the onion and celery over low heat for 15 minutes, or until soft. Add the garlic and cook for a further 2 minutes.

Meanwhile, prepare the avocado(s). Carefully cut the flesh into quarters lengthways and peel off the skin. Put three-quarters of the avocado flesh into a small bowl and mash with a fork. Cut the remaining avocado into thin slices, transfer to a bowl, sprinkle over half the lime juice to prevent discoloration and set aside.

Add the mashed avocado, the remaining lime juice and the broth to the pan with the onion and celery, bring to a simmer and cook for 5 minutes. Let cool for a few minutes, then transfer the soup to a food processor and blend until smooth. Return the soup to the pan, stir in the yoghurt and paprika and season well with salt and pepper.

The soup can be served either warm or chilled. If serving warm, gently reheat the soup, ladle into bowls, then place half the remaining avocado in the centre of each bowl of soup and garnish with the coriander. If serving cold, ladle the soup into bowls and place in the fridge until ready to serve, then add the remaining sliced avocado and garnish with the coriander.

CHICKEN, ASPARAGUS & TARRAGON SOUP

Serves 2

125 g (4 oz) asparagus spears
1 tbsp butter or coconut oil
2 celery sticks, sliced
1 leek, sliced
1 brown onion, sliced
750 ml (1¼ pints) Chicken Broth
 (*see page 142*)
1 rounded tbsp ground almonds
2 small handfuls cooked shredded
 chicken
1 tbsp chopped fresh tarragon,
 chopped (If you have to buy
 more tarragon than you need,
 chop any leftover leaves, mash
 them into butter and freeze in
 ice-cube trays)

To garnish
natural probiotic yoghurt
lemon wedges

Asparagus is a good source of prebiotic fibre but unfortunately it is not always in season. Out of season, replace the asparagus with cavalo nero.

Cut the tips off the asparagus spears to form 3-cm (1¼-inch) lengths. Roughly chop the remaining asparagus stalks.

Melt the butter or coconut oil in a large, heavy-based pan. Add the celery, leek and onion and gently sauté over low heat for 15–20 minutes until soft and translucent. Add the broth to the pan and bring to the boil, then add the chopped asparagus stalks, reduce the heat and simmer for 5 minutes. Let cool for a few minutes, then transfer the soup to a food processor and blend until smooth. Return the soup to the pan, stir in the almonds, asparagus tips and shredded chicken and simmer for 10 minutes, adding the tarragon for the last minute of cooking time.

Ladle the soup into bowls, top with a dollop of yoghurt and serve with lemon wedges to squeeze over.

LEEK & FENNEL SOUP WITH TOASTED WALNUTS

Serves 2

1 tbsp butter (or olive oil if you prefer)

2 leeks, chopped

1 small potato, diced

1 small fennel bulb, cored and chopped (reserve the leafy fronds)

1 apple, peeled and chopped

½ tsp ground turmeric

750 ml (1¼ pints) Chicken Broth (*see page 142*) or vegetable broth

sea salt and freshly ground black pepper

10 walnut halves, toasted, to garnish

Melt the butter or olive oil in a large, heavy-based pan. Add the leeks, potato and fennel and sauté over medium heat for 5 minutes. Reduce the heat to low, add the apple and turmeric, stir well and cook over low heat for 15 minutes. Pour over the broth and bring to the boil. Let cool for a few minutes, then transfer the soup to a food processor and blend until smooth. Return the soup to the pan and reheat gently. Season with salt and pepper.

Ladle the soup into bowls and sprinkle over the walnuts and fennel fronds.

This dish is ideal for alleviating bloating. Fennel is soothing and gently moving, helping to warm the body and prevent Stagnation.

CHICKEN SOUP WITH COURGETTE NOODLES

Serves 2

2 courgettes
1 tbsp olive oil
1 leek, finely sliced
2 carrots, sliced on the diagonal
1 garlic clove, crushed
750 ml (1¼ pints) Chicken Broth
   (*see page 142*)
100 g (3½ oz) cooked chicken,
   sliced
1 tsp grated lemon zest
1 large handful spinach
sea salt and freshly ground black
   pepper

Using a spiraliser fitted with the thin noodle blade, spiralise the courgettes. Alternatively, use a vegetable peeler to cut the courgettes into ribbons.

Heat the oil in a large, heavy-based pan. Add the leek and carrot and sauté over low heat for 15 minutes, or until soft, then add the garlic and cook for 1 minute more. Pour over the broth and bring to the boil. Add the chicken, bring back to the boil, then reduce the heat and simmer for 5 minutes. Add the courgette noodles and cook for 2 minutes, then stir in the lemon zest and spinach and season with salt and pepper. Remove from the heat and let stand for 5 minutes before serving.

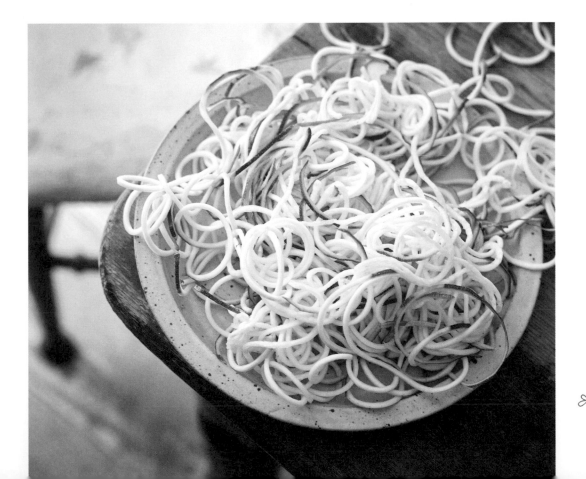

DAHL WITH ROASTED TOMATOES

Serves 4–6

375 g (12 oz) red lentils

1½ tbsp olive oil or ghee, plus extra
   for oiling the tomatoes

300 g (10 oz) cherry tomatoes

2 brown onions, chopped

1 garlic clove, crushed

2-cm (¾-inch) piece fresh ginger
   root, peeled and chopped

1 tsp garam masala

1 tsp ground turmeric

1 tsp cumin seeds

1 tsp coriander seeds

½ tsp ground nutmeg

1 tsp mustard seeds

½ tsp chopped dried chilli
   (optional)

1.2 litres (2 pints) Chicken Broth
   (*see page 142*) or vegetable broth

200 ml (7 fl oz) passata

sea salt and freshly ground black
   pepper

To garnish

natural yoghurt or kefir, to serve

1 handful fresh coriander leaves,
   chopped

6 mint leaves, shredded

Rinse the lentils under cold running water, then put them into a bowl, cover with cold water and let soak overnight.

The next day, preheat the oven to 150°C/300°F/Gas Mark 2. Rinse the lentils under cold running water and drain well.

Rub a little oil over the cherry tomatoes, then place them a roasting tin and season with salt and pepper. Bake in the oven for 45 minutes. Remove from the oven, cover with foil and set aside.

Meanwhile, heat the olive oil or ghee in a large, heavy-based pan. Add the onion and garlic and cook over low heat for 15 minutes until soft and translucent. Add the ginger and spices and cook for a couple of minutes, stirring continuously. Add the lentils and stir well to coat in the spiced oil and onions. Add the broth and passata and bring to the boil, then cover with a lid and cook over low heat for 1 hour, checking from time to time to make sure the dahl isn't drying out and adding a little more stock or water if necessary.

Ladle the dahl into bowls, place some roasted tomatoes on top, then add a dollop of yoghurt or kefir and sprinkle with the coriander and mint.

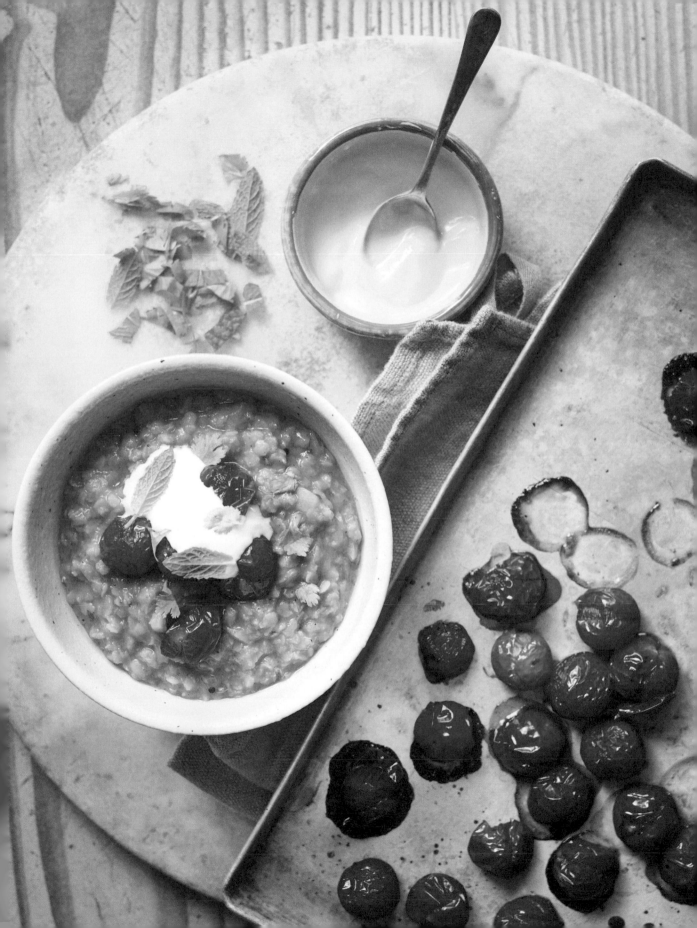

SWEET POTATO, CAVOLO NERO & ALMOND SOUP

Serves 2

1 tbsp olive oil

1 red onion, diced

1 small sweet potato, peeled and diced

2-cm (¾-inch) piece fresh root ginger, peeled and grated

500 ml (17 fl oz) Chicken Broth (*see page 142*) or vegetable broth

2 tbsp smooth almond butter

80 g (3 oz) cavolo nero, shredded

2 tbsp chopped fresh flatleaf parsley, to garnish

Heat the oil in a large, heavy-based pan. Add the onion and cook over low heat for 15 minutes. Add the sweet potato, ginger and broth and cook for 10 minutes more. Let cool for a few minutes, then transfer the soup to a food processor and blend until smooth. Return the soup to the pan.

Put a little of the soup into a small bowl with the almond butter and whisk together. Set aside.

Add the cavolo nero to the pan with the soup, cover with a lid and cook over low heat for 10 minutes. Stir in the almond butter mixture just before you are ready to serve.

Ladle the soup into bowls and garnish with the parsley.

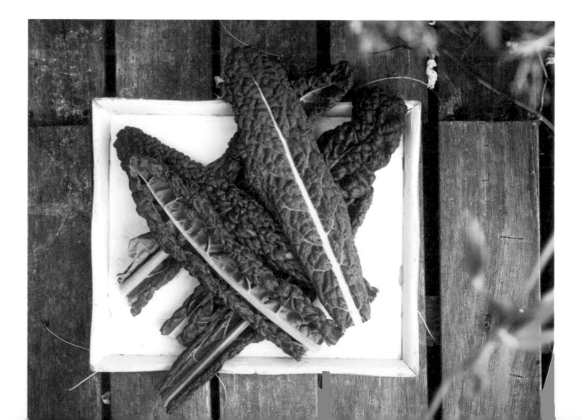

LENTIL & LEAFY GREENS SOUP

Serves 2

150 g (5 oz) red lentils
1 tbsp olive oil or coconut oil
1 red onion, chopped
1 leek, thinly sliced
1 celery stick, thinly sliced
1 garlic clove, crushed
½ tsp ground cumin
½ tsp ground coriander
¼ tsp ground turmeric
600 ml (1 pint) Chicken Broth (*see page 142*) or vegetable broth
100 g (3½ oz) leafy greens, such as Swiss chard, cavolo nero or spinach, shredded
sea salt and freshly ground black pepper

To garnish
15 g (½ oz) fresh coriander
grated zest of ½ unwaxed lemon

Rinse the lentils under cold running water, then put them into a bowl, cover with cold water and let soak overnight.

The next day, rinse the lentils under cold running water and drain well. Place the lentils in a large pan and cover with cold water. Bring to the boil, then reduce the heat and simmer for 20 minutes. Drain well.

Meanwhile, heat the olive or coconut oil in a large, heavy-based pan. Add the onion, leek and celery and sauté over low heat for 15 minutes, adding the garlic 2 minutes before the end of the cooking time. Stir in the spices and remove from the heat.

Transfer the onion mixture to a food processor, add half the lentils and the broth and blend until smooth. Return the soup to the pan, add the leafy greens and bring to the boil, then reduce the heat and simmer for 5 minutes. Add the remaining lentils and cook for 5 minutes more. Season with salt and pepper.

Ladle the soup into bowls and garnish with the fresh coriander and lemon zest.

CHICORY, PRESERVED LEMON & SPELT SOUP

Serves 2

1 tbsp olive oil

1 small onion, thinly sliced

1 celery stick, thinly sliced

600 ml (1 pint) Chicken Broth (*see page 142*) or vegetable broth

1 head red chicory, chopped into 4-cm (1¾-inch) pieces

100 g (3½ oz) cooked spelt

½ small preserved lemon, flesh removed and rind finely diced

1 small dried chilli, crumbled (optional)

sea salt and freshly ground black pepper

To garnish

2 tbsp crème fraîche

1 handful flatleaf parsley, chopped

Spelt is an ancient grain that has a distinctive nutty flavour. If gluten is tolerated, spelt is a gentle and nourishing alternative to conventional wheat.

Heat the oil in a large, heavy-based pan. Add the onion and celery and sauté over low heat for 15 minutes. Pour over the broth and bring to the boil, then add the chicory, reduce the heat and simmer for 10 minutes. Stir in the spelt, preserved lemon rind and chilli, if using. Season with salt and pepper.

Ladle the soup into bowls, add dollops of crème fraîche and garnish with the parsley.

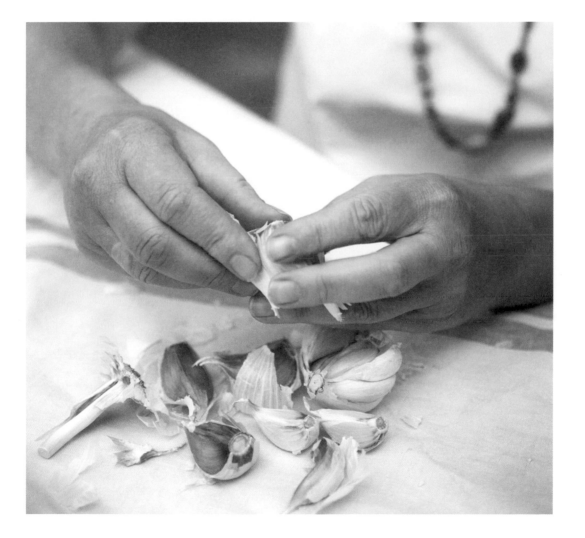

Condiments

NATURALLY FERMENTED SAUERKRAUT

Makes 1 x 500-ml (17-fl oz) jar

1 head white cabbage, finely
   shredded
1½ tbsp sea salt

Put the cabbage into a large bowl and lightly sprinkle with the salt. Using your hands, massage, squeeze and knead the cabbage for about 10 minutes to help it release its natural juices – the cabbage will become watery and limp.

Transfer the cabbage with its juices to a sterilised jar (*see page 139*) or traditional fermentation crock. Pack the cabbage in tightly and press down really hard to eliminate air bubbles. If necessary, add some weights to make sure the cabbage is submerged in its liquid. Seal the jar or crock.

Store in a cool, dark place at room temperature for 3–5 days while it ferments, opening the lid once a day to release any built up-pressure (burping!). When the vegetables are bubbly and tangy the kraut is ready. You can now transfer it to the fridge, where it will continue to ferment and develop in flavour over the next few weeks.

You can eat the sauerkraut immediately or store it for up to 6 months in the fridge.

GOLDEN KRAUT

Makes 1 x 500-ml (17-fl oz) jar

1 Chinese leaf cabbage (remove the outer leaves but keep a couple aside), finely shredded

2 large carrots, grated

1 mooli (white radish), grated (you can replace this with a thumb-sized piece of peeled and grated fresh root ginger if you prefer)

1½ tbsp sea salt

1 tsp grated fresh turmeric root

1 tbsp caraway seeds

Put the cabbage, carrots, mooli and salt into a large bowl. Using your hands, massage, squeeze and knead the vegetables for about 10 minutes to help them release their natural juices – the vegetables will become watery and limp. Add the turmeric and caraway and mix well.

Transfer the vegetables with their juices to a sterilised jar (*see page 139*). Pack the vegetables in tightly and press down really hard to eliminate air bubbles. Place the reserved outer leaves of the cabbage on top and press down firmly to make sure the vegetables are submerged in their liquid.

Store in a cool, dark place at room temperature for 3–5 days while it ferments, opening the lid once a day to release any built up-pressure (burping!). When the vegetables are bubbly and tangy the kraut is ready. You can now transfer it to the fridge, where it will continue to ferment and develop in flavour over the next few weeks.

You can eat the kraut immediately or store it for up to 6 months in the fridge.

Turmeric has powerful anti-inflammatory properties and turns the kraut a gorgeous sunshine yellow.

GREEN KRAUT

Makes 1 x 500-ml (17–fl oz) jar

3 heads spring greens, finely
    shredded
10 wild garlic, finely shredded
3 spring onions, finely sliced
1½ tbsp sea salt
1½ tbsp dried seaweed flakes

Cruciferous vegetables (including broccoli, kale, cauliflower and cabbage) contain goitrogenic substances that have the potential to affect hormone function and thyroid medication. These foods are fine when consumed after they have been cooked as cooking inactivates the goitrogens. The effect may also be offset by adequate iodine (e.g. seafood) and selenium (e.g. seafood and sunflower seeds) intake. When making sauerkraut add a little dried seaweed as an iodine source to counteract the intake of goitrogenic substances from the raw greens.

Put the spring greens, garlic leaves and spring onions into a large bowl and sprinkle over the salt and seaweed. Using your hands, massage, squeeze and knead the vegetables for about 10 minutes to help them release their natural juices – the vegetables will become watery and limp.

Transfer the vegetables with their juices to a sterilised jar (*see page 139*). Pack the vegetables in tightly and press down really hard to eliminate air bubbles. Place some weights on top and press down firmly to make sure the vegetables are submerged in their liquid.

Store in a cool, dark place at room temperature for 3–5 days while it ferments, opening the lid once a day to release any built up-pressure (burping!). When the vegetables are bubbly and tangy the kraut is ready. You can now transfer it to the fridge, where it will continue to ferment and develop in flavour over the next few weeks.

You can eat the kraut immediately or store it for up to 6 months in the fridge.

WHEY & KEFIR CHEESE

Makes 300 ml (½ pint) whey and 125 g (4 oz) kefir cheese

500 ml (17 fl oz) kefir

Whey is what remains when the fats and solids are removed from milk. Whey is often used as a starter culture for fermenting vegetables but it has many other culinary uses: enriching stocks, tenderising meat, as a cooking liquid for pulses and wholegrains, as a base for alcohol (even being used as a trendy cocktail ingredient) and as a refreshing drink on its own.

It is easy to make whey at home from either kefir or natural live yoghurt, and the method has the added benefit that the leftover milk fats and solids form a delicious soft cheese.

Line a small bowl with a large piece of cheesecloth. Carefully pour the kefir into the prepared bowl, bring up the edges of the cheesecloth to form a bag and secure with rubber bands.

Using kitchen string, suspend the bag over a bowl and leave overnight to drain. It is ready when the bag stops dripping and all the whey is collected in the bowl.

Store the whey in a sterilised jar (*see page 139*) in the fridge until you are ready to use. It can be stored for up to 6 months in the fridge.

Unwrap the cheesecloth and transfer the kefir cheese to an airtight container. It can be stored in the fridge for up to a week but is best eaten within a couple of days.

IDEAS FOR USING KEFIR CHEESE

Mix the cheese with chopped herbs and extra virgin to make a herby soft cheese.

Stuff mini sweet peppers with the cheese.

Serve it with roasted beetroot.

Spread it on toasted sourdough.

LACTO-FERMENTED SALSA

Makes 4 x 375-ml (13-fl oz) jars

1.2 kg (2½ lb) small tomatoes,
  quartered or diced
2 tbsp sea salt
1 large bunch fresh coriander,
  finely chopped
1 red onion, diced
5 garlic cloves, thinly sliced
1 red chilli, finely sliced
4 tbsp Whey (*see page 163*)
juice of 1 lime

Lacto-fermentation is a natural process that allows for the growth of microbes. The microbes eat the vegetables' sugars and produce lactic acid, inhibiting the growth of harmful microbes. Lacto-fermentation preserves food, increases the nutritional content and digestibility and provides microbes.

Put the tomatoes into a large bowl and sprinkle over the salt. Using your hands, squeeze the tomatoes until they have a soupy consistency. Add the remaining ingredients and mix well.

Transfer to sterilised jars (*see page 139*) and seal immediately. Store in a cool, dark place at room temperature for 3–5 days until the mixture is bubbly and fermented, opening the lid once a day to release any built up-pressure. Taste after 3 days and if you are happy with the flavour – it should taste tangy and slightly effervescent – transfer to the fridge. It can be stored for up to 6 months in the fridge.

WALNUT TARATOR SAUCE

Serves 6

60 g (2½ oz) walnuts

50 g (2 oz) brown sourdough breadcrumbs

1 garlic clove, crushed

1½ tbsp white balsamic vinegar

1 tbsp fresh lemon juice

150 ml (¼ pint) extra virgin olive oil

sea salt and freshly ground black pepper

This sauce is traditionally served with fish or roasted vegetables or used as a dip. The walnuts can be replaced with lightly toasted almonds or hazelnuts.

Heat a small, dry frying pan over a medium heat and add the walnuts. Stir frequently until the walnuts start to brown and smell toasted, about 5 minutes. Set aside to cool for a few minutes.

Put the walnuts, breadcrumbs, garlic, balsamic vinegar, lemon juice and a pinch of salt into a food processor and blend until smooth, gradually adding the oil in a thin stream until you have a thick and creamy sauce. If you prefer your sauce to have a thinner consistency, add a little extra oil. Season to taste with salt and pepper.

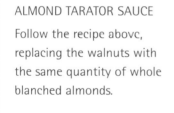

ALMOND TARATOR SAUCE

Follow the recipe above, replacing the walnuts with the same quantity of whole blanched almonds.

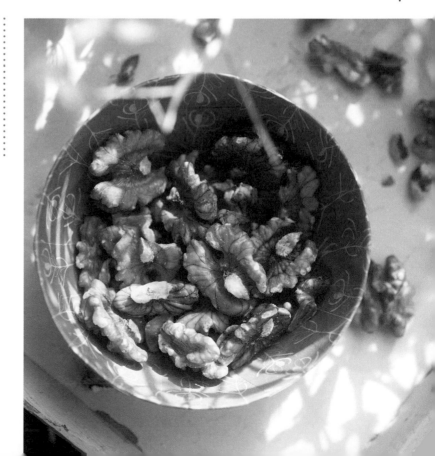

WALNUT & BEETROOT PESTO

Makes 375 g (12 oz)

3 tbsp olive oil
2 raw beetroot, grated
50 g (2 oz) walnuts
1 garlic clove, crushed
50 g (2 oz) flatleaf parsley
sea salt and freshly ground black
   pepper

Heat 1 tablespoon of oil in a frying pan. Add the beetroot and sauté over low heat for 10 minutes, or until softened.

Put half the beetroot into a food processor, add the remaining oil and the walnuts, garlic and parsley and blend until smooth. Alternatively, use a handheld blender to purée the ingredients.

Transfer the pesto to a bowl, add the remaining beetroot, season with salt and pepper and mix well.

This pesto will keep in an airtight container in the fridge for a couple of days or it can be spooned into ice-cube trays and frozen.

WALNUT & ROCKET PESTO

Makes 375 g (12 oz)

70 g (2¾ oz) wild rocket
60 g (2½ oz) walnuts, toasted
50 g (2 oz) basil
1 small garlic clove, crushed
100 g (3½ oz) Parmesan cheese
   or vegetarian Parmesan-style
   cheese, grated
1 tsp grated unwaxed lemon zest
2 tbsp extra virgin olive oil
sea salt and freshly ground black
   pepper

Whiz all the ingredients in a food processor, or purée with a handheld blender, until the mixture is smooth.

This pesto will keep in an airtight container in the fridge for a couple of days or it can be spooned into ice-cube trays and frozen.

BRAZIL NUT & ROCKET PESTO
Follow the recipe above, replacing the walnuts with 60 g (2½ oz) toasted brazil nuts.

NETTLE PESTO

Makes 100 g (3½ oz)

2 tbsp nettle leaf powder
4 tbsp extra virgin olive oil
1 garlic clove, peeled
2 tbsp pumpkin seeds
1 tbsp pine nuts
pinch of sea salt

This unusual pesto can be enjoyed in so many ways: whisk some together with a little oil to make a salad dressing or spread it on toasted sourdough bread.

Whiz all the ingredients in a food processor, or purée with a handheld blender, until the mixture is smooth.

This pesto will keep in an airtight container in the fridge for up to 3 days or it can be spooned into ice-cube trays and frozen.

CHESTNUT & HERB PESTO

Makes 375 g (12 oz)

100 g (3½ oz) vacuum-packed
   chestnuts
1 small garlic clove, crushed
12 large sage leaves
25 g (1 oz) flatleaf parsley
2 tbsp extra virgin olive oil

Whiz all the ingredients in a food processor, or purée with a handheld blender, until the mixture is coarsely chopped.

This pesto will keep in an airtight container in the fridge for up to 1 week or it can be spooned into ice-cube trays and frozen.

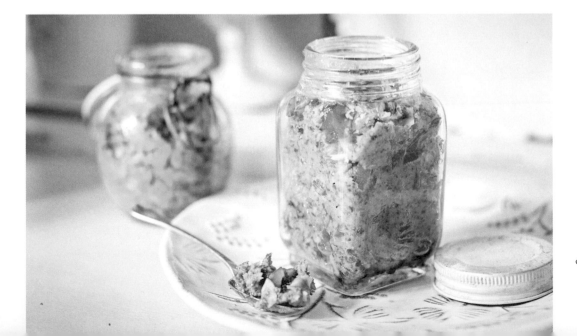

NUT, SPICE & SEED MIX

Makes 2 x 375-ml (13-fl oz) jars

100 g (3½ oz) hazelnuts
50 g (2 oz) brazil nuts
2 tbsp cumin seeds
3 tbsp coriander seeds
3 tbsp pumpkin seeds
2 tbsp black sesame seeds
2 tsp fennel seeds
2 tbsp white peppercorns
1 tbsp ground turmeric
1 tsp paprika
1 tsp sea salt

THRIFTY TIP

I like to make enough of this condiment so that I have some for myself and can also fill a couple of spice jars to give to friends, but feel free to halve the quantities for this recipe if you prefer.

This fragrant and nourishing mixture of nuts, spices and seeds is based on an Egyptian dukkah – the word is derived from the Arabic 'dakka' (meaning 'to crush'). Traditionally dukkah is eaten by dipping some bread first in olive oil and then in the spice mix. It is a versatile storecupboard ingredient that can be used to enrich and season many dishes, such as roasted vegetables, salads, pasta and seasonal greens, or it can be stirred through yoghurt or sprinkled over poached eggs for breakfast.

Preheat the oven to 200°C/400°C/Gas Mark 6.

Spread out the nuts on a baking sheet and bake in the oven for 5 minutes, or until they have darkened and their aroma is released. Let cool and then rub the nuts between your fingertips to loosen their skins. Remove and discard the skins.

Heat a dry, cast-iron frying pan, add the cumin seeds and roast over medium heat for a couple of minutes to release their aroma. Transfer to a bowl and set aside. Repeat with the coriander seeds, followed by the pumpkin seeds, then the sesame seeds, then the fennel seeds, and finally the peppercorns.

Put all ingredients into a food processor or nut grinder and process until coarsely chopped. Alternatively, if you'd like the mixture to retain more of its crunch, use a mortar and pestle to grind the mixture to your desired consistency. Store in an airtight container in a cool, dark place.

SPICY PUMPKIN SEEDS

Makes 1 x 375-ml (13-fl oz) jar

⅛ tsp cayenne pepper
¼ tsp smoked paprika
1 tsp dried seaweed flakes
½ tbsp olive oil
100 g (3½ oz) pumpkin seeds
sea salt, for sprinkling

Mix together the cayenne, paprika and seaweed in a shallow dish.

Heat the oil in a frying pan. Add the pumpkin seeds and cook over medium heat for 2–3 minutes, stirring continuously, until the seeds are warm and coated in the oil.

Transfer the seeds to the dish with the spice mixture and toss well to coat. Spread out the seeds on a baking sheet or large plate and sprinkle with a little salt. Let cool.

The seeds can be stored in an airtight container for up to 1 week.

SARDINE PÂTÉ

Serves 2 for lunch or 4 as a starter

2 x 120-g (4-oz) cans sardines in olive oil
juice of ½ small unwaxed lemon, plus 1 tsp grated lemon zest
50 g (2 oz) butter
1 garlic clove, crushed
5 g (¼ oz) dill, chopped, plus extra to garnish
¼ tsp cayenne pepper
¼ tsp sea salt
¼tsp black pepper

Choose good-quality tinned sardines in olive oil. Tinned sardines are a good source of calcium as you are able to eat the soft, edible bones.

Put all the ingredients into a food processor (including the oil from the sardines) and blend until smooth. If you prefer a coarser texture, blend for a little less time.

Spoon the pâté into a small serving bowl and garnish with a little extra dill. Cover with foil and chill in the fridge for a couple of hours before serving. The pâté will keep for a couple of days in the fridge.

CHICKPEA & DATE HOUMOUS

Serves 2–3

50 g (2 oz) black sesame seeds
4 tbsp olive oil
1 x 400-g (13-oz) can chickpeas,
    drained
4 Medjool dates, pitted
1 small garlic clove, crushed
juice of ½–1 lemon
sea salt

Heat a dry frying pan, add the sesame seeds and roast over medium heat for 2–3 minutes, shaking the pan or stirring occasionally, until fragrant.

If you like your houmous to have texture, jump straight to the next step. If you prefer a smooth houmous, put the sesame seeds into a food processor, add half the oil and process until smooth, then set aside.

Put the chickpeas, dates, garlic, 2 tablespoons of lemon juice and the oil (or remaining oil if you've already made the sesame seeds paste) and blend until smooth.

Transfer the houmous to a bowl and stir in the sesame seeds or sesame seed paste.

Season to taste with salt and lemon juice. This houmous will keep in the fridge for up to 3 days.

Fish, meat & poultry

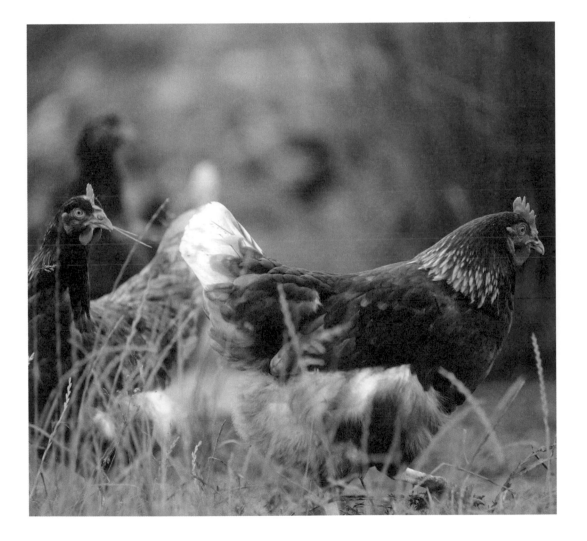

MOROCCAN-SPICED CHICKEN LIVERS

Serves 2

1½ tsp ground coriander

¼ tsp ground cinnamon

1 tsp ground cumin

1 tsp smoked paprika

pinch of cayenne pepper

1½ tbsp chickpea flour

1 tbsp olive oil

300 g (10 oz) chicken livers, cut
into bite-sized pieces

knob of butter

sea salt and freshly ground black
pepper

1 tbsp chopped fresh coriander,
to garnish

Mix together the spices, flour and oil in a bowl and season with salt and pepper. Add the chicken livers and toss thoroughly to coat the livers with the spice mixture. Let marinate in the fridge for 30 minutes.

Heat the butter in a frying pan. Add the chicken livers and cook over high heat for 2 minutes on each side.

Serve immediately, garnished with the coriander.

I know that liver isn't everyone's favourite ingredient but I encourage you to try and add some to your diet, especially post-menstrually. Liver is Blood-nourishing and it warms the body.

PORK & CHICKEN LIVER MEATBALLS WITH CREAMY POLENTA

Serves 2

For the meatballs
300 g (10 oz) pork mince
100 g (3½ oz) chicken livers,
   chopped finely
1 tbsp fennel seeds
pinch of chilli flakes
1 large egg
1 garlic clove, crushed
1 tbsp olive oil
sea salt and freshly ground black
   pepper
10 g (½ oz) chopped flatleaf
   parsley, to garnish

For the sauce
1½ tsp olive oil
1 red onion, finely chopped
1 x 400-g (13-oz) carton chopped
   tomatoes
1 tbsp red wine vinegar
15 g (½ oz) chopped flatleaf
   parsley

For the polenta
100 g (3½ oz) instant polenta
   (cornmeal)
15 g (½ oz) butter
15 g (½ oz) Parmesan cheese,
   grated

First make the meatballs. Put the pork, chicken livers, fennel seeds, chilli, egg and garlic into a bowl and mix well. Season with salt and pepper. Using your hands, divide the mixture into 6 portions and roll each one into a ball that is a little larger than a golf ball. If you have the time, transfer the meatballs to a plate and let chill in the fridge for a couple of hours to allow the meatballs to firm up. You can cook them immediately but they will be more fragile.

Heat the oil in a large, heavy-based pan. Add the meatballs and cook over medium heat for about 5 minutes, turning from time to time, until golden brown on each side. Remove with a slotted spoon and set aside.

Now make the sauce. In the same pan, heat the oil, then add the onion and sauté over low heat for 10 minutes, or until soft and translucent. Add the tomatoes and vinegar and bring to the boil, then reduce the heat slightly and allow the sauce to bubble for 10 minutes. Add the meatballs and parsley, cover with a lid and cook over low heat for 25 minutes. Remove the lid and cook for 5 minutes more.

Meanwhile, make the polenta. Bring 500 ml (17 fl oz) water to the boil in a pan. Reduce the heat to low and slowly pour in the polenta in a thin stream, whisking all the time. Cook over low heat for 5 minutes, stirring from time to time. Remove from the heat and stir in the butter and Parmesan. Season with salt and pepper

Divide the meatballs and tomato sauce between plates, garnish with the parsley and serve with the polenta.

STIR-FRIED KIDNEYS WITH GINGER & SESAME

Serves 2

4 lambs' kidneys

2 tbsp olive oil or coconut oil

2-cm (¾-inch) piece fresh root
ginger, peeled and finely chopped

3 spring onions, sliced on the
diagonal

125 g (4 oz) tenderstem broccoli

8 shiitake mushrooms

1 red chilli, seeded and chopped

1 garlic clove, crushed

1 tbsp soy sauce

1 tbsp Shaoxing rice wine

cooked rice or buckwheat noodles,
to serve

To garnish

2 tbsp chopped fresh coriander

1 tbsp black sesame seeds

First prepare the kidneys. Cut them in half and rinse thoroughly under cold running water. Remove the outer membrane. Using a pair of scissors, snip out the tight white core. Cut the livers into 5-mm (¼-inch) slices.

Heat 1 tablespoon of oil in a large frying pan or wok. Add the kidneys and stir fry over high heat for 3 minutes. Remove the kidneys from the pan or wok and set aside.

Heat the remaining oil in the pan or wok, then add the ginger and spring onions and stir fry for 5 minutes, or until the ginger has darkened. Add the broccoli, mushrooms, chilli and garlic and stir fry for 5 minutes, then pour over the soy sauce and Shaoxing rice wine and stir fry for 2 minutes more. Return the kidneys to the pan and stir fry for a couple of minutes until heated through.

Divide the stir fry between dishes, garnish with the coriander and sesame seeds and serve with cooked rice or buckwheat noodles.

KIDNEYS & MUSHROOMS IN A CREAMY MUSTARD SAUCE WITH PUY LENTILS

Serves 2

6 lambs' kidneys
25 g (1 oz) butter
1 red onion, finely diced
150 g (5 oz) chestnut mushrooms,
    thickly sliced
1 tbsp Dijon mustard
80 g (3 oz) crème fraîche
20 g (¾ oz) flatleaf parsley,
    chopped

For the Puy lentils

1 tbsp olive oil
1 shallot, chopped
1 celery stick, finely diced
100 g (3½ oz) Puy lentils
375 ml (13 fl oz) Chicken Broth (*see
    page 142*)
1 sprig thyme, leaves only
glug of extra virgin olive oil
sea salt and freshly ground black
    pepper

First make the Puy lentils. Heat the oil in a pan, then add the shallot and celery and cook over low heat for 10 minutes. Stir in the lentils to coat in the oil. Pour over the broth, add the thyme and bring to the boil. Reduce the heat and simmer for 15–20 minutes until the lentils are al dente. Drain well and transfer to a bowl. Drizzle over a glug of extra virgin olive oil, stir gently and season with salt and pepper.

Meanwhile, prepare the kidneys. Cut them in half and rinse thoroughly under cold running water. Remove the outer membrane. Using a pair of scissors, snip out the tight white core. Cut the livers into 5-mm (¼-inch) slices.

Heat the butter in a frying pan. Add the onion and sauté over low heat for 10 minutes, or until softened. Add the kidneys and cook over high heat for 1 minute, stirring continuously, then add the mushrooms and cook over medium–high heat for 4–5 minutes until lightly browned. Stir in the mustard and crème fraîche and cook until the sauce is bubbling. Stir in the parsley and season with salt and pepper.

Divide the kidneys and mushrooms between dishes and serve with the Puy lentils.

GRILLED MACKEREL WITH PROBIOTIC KOHLRABI & FENNEL COLESLAW

Serves 2

2 whole mackerel, cleaned, scaled
and gutted, with heads and tails
left on
olive oil

**For the kohlrabi & fennel
coleslaw**

100 g (3½ oz) natural probiotic
yoghurt
1 small garlic clove, crushed
1 tsp apple cider vinegar
1 fennel bulb, finely sliced (reserve
the leafy fronds)
1 kohlrabi, finely sliced
2 carrots, coarsely grated
2 spring onions, finely sliced
lengthways
1 tbsp pumpkin seeds
1 tbsp walnuts
sea salt and freshly ground black
pepper

First make the coleslaw. Make a dressing by whisking together the yoghurt, garlic and vinegar in a bowl, then season with a little salt and pepper. Put the remaining ingredients, except for the fennel fronds, into a large bowl, pour over the dressing and stir together gently. Garnish with the fennel fronds.

Preheat the grill to high. Alternatively, light the barbecue and wait until it is hot and ready to cook over.

Season the mackerel with salt and pepper. Rub a little oil over the fillets and then lay them, skin-side up, on the grill pan.

Place the fish under the grill or on the barbecue and cook for a few minutes on each side until the flesh is opaque and the skin has crisped.

Serve the mackerel with the coleslaw.

ROASTED SARDINES WITH TOMATO, ONION & POMEGRANATE

Serves 2

2 tbsp olive oil, plus extra for greasing
1 unwaxed lemon
½ red onion, finely diced
½ tsp fennel seeds, toasted
1 garlic clove, sliced
1 fennel bulb, thinly sliced
10 cherry tomatoes, halved
4 whole sardines, cleaned and gutted
seeds from ½ pomegranate (you can use the rest of the seeds for breakfast)
sea salt and freshly ground black pepper
1 tbsp chopped fresh flatleaf parsley, to garnish
cooked freekah, quinoa or other wholegrains, to serve (optional)

Preheat the oven to 180°C/350°C/Gas Mark 4. Grease a roasting tin with oil

Cut the lemon in half. Cut one half of the lemon into thin slices. Grate the zest of the other half of the lemon and reserve the juice.

In a small bowl, mix together the onion, fennel seeds, garlic, lemon juice and zest and 1 tablespoon of oil. Season with salt and pepper.

Spread the fennel slices over a small baking sheet and drizzle over the remaining oil. Arrange the lemon slices and tomatoes on top of the fennel.

Stuff the cavities of the sardines with some of the onion mixture and place in the prepared roasting tin. Scatter any remaining onion mixture over and around the sardines and sprinkle over the pomegranate seeds. Roast in the oven for 10–15 minutes until the fish is cooked through.

Garnish the sardines with parsley and serve with cooked freekah, quinoa or other wholegrains, if liked. The fish can be served hot or at room temperature.

BEEF, BROCCOLI & QUINOA STIR FRY

Serves 2

80 g (3 oz) quinoa
juice of ½ lime
2 tbsp tamari soy sauce
1 tbsp toasted sesame oil
1 tsp brown rice vinegar
1 tbsp coconut oil
2.5-cm (1-inch) piece fresh root
  ginger, peeled and grated
2 garlic cloves, crushed
4 spring onions, cut in half and
  then sliced lengthways
150 g (5 oz) tenderstem broccoli,
  cut in half lengthways
2 sirloin steaks, cut into 5-mm
  (¼-inch) strips
100 g (3½ oz) bean sprouts
2 tsp black sesame seeds
cos lettuce leaves, to serve

Cook the quinoa in a large pan of boiling water according to the packet instructions until tender, then drain well.

In a small bowl, whisk together the lime juice, soy sauce, sesame oil and vinegar and set aside.

Heat the coconut oil in a large frying pan or wok. Add the ginger and cook over medium heat until it is darkened but not charred. Add the garlic, spring onions and broccoli and stir fry over medium heat for 5 minutes. Add the steak and stir fry for 3 minutes. Add the bean sprouts and stir fry over high heat for 1 minute more, or longer if you prefer your beef more well done. Add the quinoa and sesame seeds, pour over the dressing and mix well.

To serve, place a couple of lettuce leaves on each plate and spoon the stir fry into them.

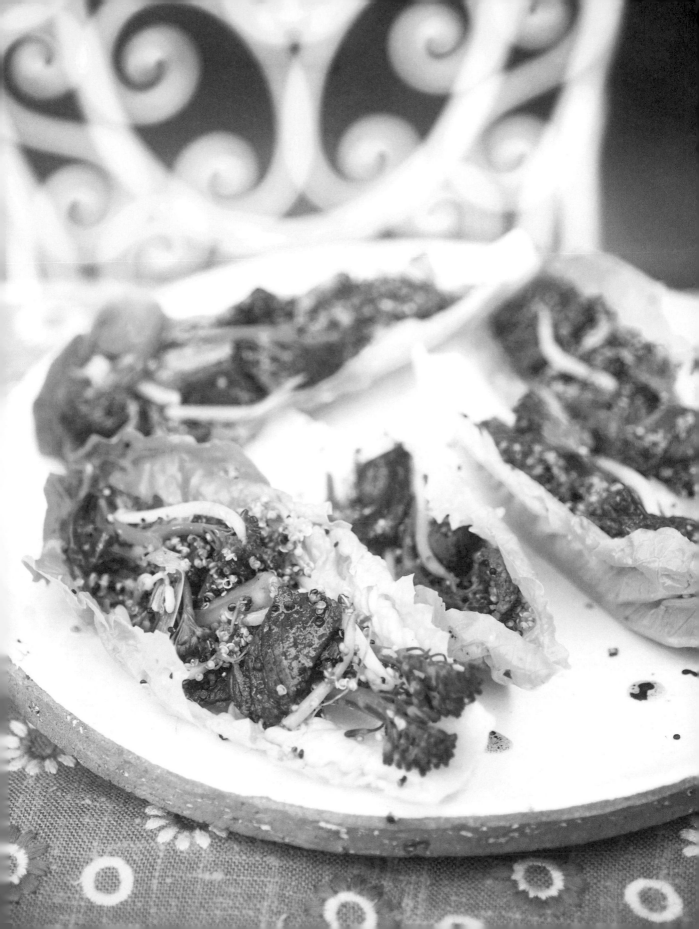

SAFFRON FISH & VEGETABLE STEW

Serves 2

1 tbsp coconut oil or olive oil
1 small bulb fennel, diced
1 carrot, grated
1 small sweet potato, cut into small
    dice
1 leek, thinly sliced
250–300 ml (8 fl oz–½ pint)
    Chicken Broth (*see page 142*)
a few saffron threads
1 tsp dried seaweed flakes
    (optional)
200 g (7 oz) firm white fish
sea salt and freshly ground black
    pepper
lemon wedges, to serve

Heat the coconut or olive oil in a wide, heavy-based pan. Add the fennel, carrot, sweet potato and leek and sauté over low heat for 10 minutes. Pour over the broth, add the saffron strands and bring to the boil, then reduce the heat and cook over low heat for another 10 minutes.

Sprinkle over the seaweed flakes, if using, and lay the fish on top of the broth and vegetables. Cover with a lid and cook over low heat until the fish is cooked through and flakes apart, about 10–15 minutes, depending on the thickness of the fish. Season to taste with salt and pepper.

Serve the stew with the lemon wedges to squeeze over.

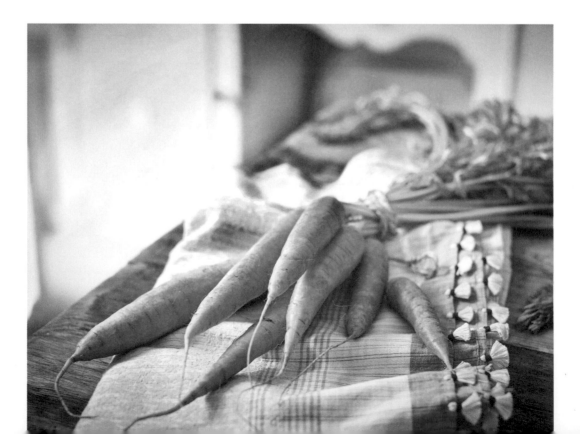

BEEF SHIN & PUMPKIN STEW

Serves 2–3

2 tbsp olive oil

350 g (11½ oz) beef shin, diced

1 large red onion, sliced

1 celery stick, sliced

1 garlic clove, crushed

2 anchovy fillets preserved in oil, drained (optional – they add a savoury taste)

½ small butternut squash, peeled, seeded and diced

200 ml (7 fl oz) passata

pinch of cayenne pepper

1 bay leaf

1 large thyme sprig, leaves only

400 ml (14 fl oz) Chicken Broth (see page 142)

sea salt and freshly ground black pepper

Preheat the oven to 150°C/300°C/Gas Mark 2.

Heat 1 tablespoon of oil in a large, ovenproof casserole. Add the beef and cook over medium heat for 5 minutes, turning occasionally, or until and browned all over. Remove the beef from the casserole and set aside.

Add the remaining oil to the casserole. Add the onion and sauté over low heat for 15 minutes, then add the celery, garlic and anchovies and cook for 2 minutes more, stirring continuously to break up the fish. Add the butternut squash and stir well before adding the passata, cayenne, bay leaf and thyme. Return the beef to the casserole, pour over the broth, season with salt and pepper and bring to a simmer. Cover the casserole with a sheet of baking paper, letting it rest in the surface, then cover with a lid and bake in the oven for 3–4 hours until the meat is tender.

The beef shin for this melt-in-the-mouth stew is slow cooked until it is so tender that it can be broken up with a spoon. Cooking increases the bioavailability of the lycopene from the tomatoes and the beta-carotene from the butternut squash.

ROASTED BONE MARROW WITH SHALLOT & PARSLEY SALAD

Serves 2

2 long marrow bones, sliced
lengthways (ask your butcher
to do this)
toasted sourdough, to serve

For the shallot & parsley salad
1 tbsp butter
1 banana shallot, finely diced
2 large handfuls flatleaf parsley
leaves, roughly chopped
grated zest of ½ unwaxed lemon
a drizzle of extra virgin olive oil
sea salt and freshly ground black
pepper

Preheat the oven to 220°C/425°C/Gas Mark 7.

Place the bones, cut-side up, in an ovenproof dish. Bake in the oven for 15–20 minutes until the marrow is bubbling slightly and has begun to come away from the bones.

Meanwhile, make the salad. Melt the butter in a small frying pan, add the shallot and cook over medium heat for 2–3 minutes until softened. Add the parsley and lemon zest and cook for 1 minute more. Remove from the heat and season with salt and pepper. Drizzle over a little oil and toss well to loosen the salad.

Scoop out the bone marrow and spread it on toasted sourdough. Divide between serving plates and accompany with the salad.

'Like treats like.' Bone marrow is a wonderful Jing tonic – the best!

TROUT WITH PRESERVED LEMON, SULTANAS & ALMONDS

Serves 2

2 rainbow trout fillets, about 140 g
(4½ oz) each, cut into bite-sized
pieces
pinch of cayenne pepper
1 tbsp olive oil
6 spring onions, thinly sliced
1 carrot, diced
1 preserved lemon, flesh removed
and rind finely diced
4 dates, pitted and finely chopped
250 ml (8 fl oz) Chicken Broth (*see
page 142*)
sea salt and freshly ground black
pepper
cooked brown rice, quinoa or
buckwheat, to serve

To garnish
2 tbsp chopped fresh coriander
1 tbsp flaked almonds, toasted

Season the trout fillets with salt, pepper and cayenne
pepper. Set aside.

Heat the oil in a large frying pan, add the spring onions and
carrot and sauté over low heat for 15 minutes, or until soft.
Add the preserved lemon rind, dates and broth and simmer
for 10 minutes. Add the trout and cook over medium–high
heat for 10 minutes. Season with salt and pepper

Divide the fish between plates, garnish with the coriander
and almonds and serve with cooked brown rice, quinoa
or buckwheat.

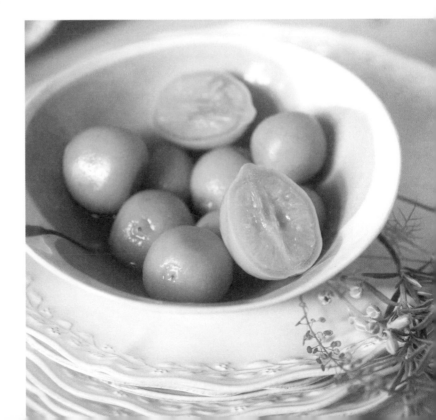

ALMOND-CRUSTED SALMON WITH CAULIFLOWER PURÉE

Serves 2

4 tbsp whole blanched almonds
1 tsp dried seaweed flakes
  (optional)
2 salmon fillets, about 140 g
  (4½ oz) each
juice of ½ lemon
2 tsp honey
sea salt and freshly ground black
  pepper

For the cauliflower purée
1 small cauliflower
200 ml (7 fl oz) Chicken Broth
  (*see page 142*)
1 tsp thyme leaves
1 generous knob of butter

WALNUT-CRUSTED SALMON

Follow the recipe above,
replacing the whole almonds
with the same quantity of
walnut halves.

Preheat the oven to 180°C/350°C/Gas Mark 4.

Using a mortar and pestle, coarsely crush the almonds, then add the seaweed flakes, if using, and season with salt and pepper

Place 2 large sheets of foil on the work counter. Put a salmon fillet in the centre of each piece of foil. Squeeze the lemon juice over the fish. Smear a teaspoon of honey over the top of each piece of salmon and then press the crushed nuts on top of the fish to form a crust. Wrap the foil around the sides of the fish, leaving the top open so the crust can toast in the oven. Bake in the oven for 20–25 minutes until the salmon is cooked through.

Meanwhile, make the cauliflower purée. Discard the tough outer leaves and then cut the smaller leaves into pieces. Break the cauliflower into florets and roughly chop the stalk. Bring the broth to the boil in a large pan, then add the cauliflower and thyme, and cook over low heat for 10–15 minutes until the cauliflower is tender. Transfer to a food processor and blend until smooth. Return to the pan, stir in the butter and cook over low heat until heated through. Season well with salt and pepper.

Divide the cauliflower purée between plates. Take the salmon out of the parcels and place on top of the cauliflower purée. Season with a little extra pepper, if liked.

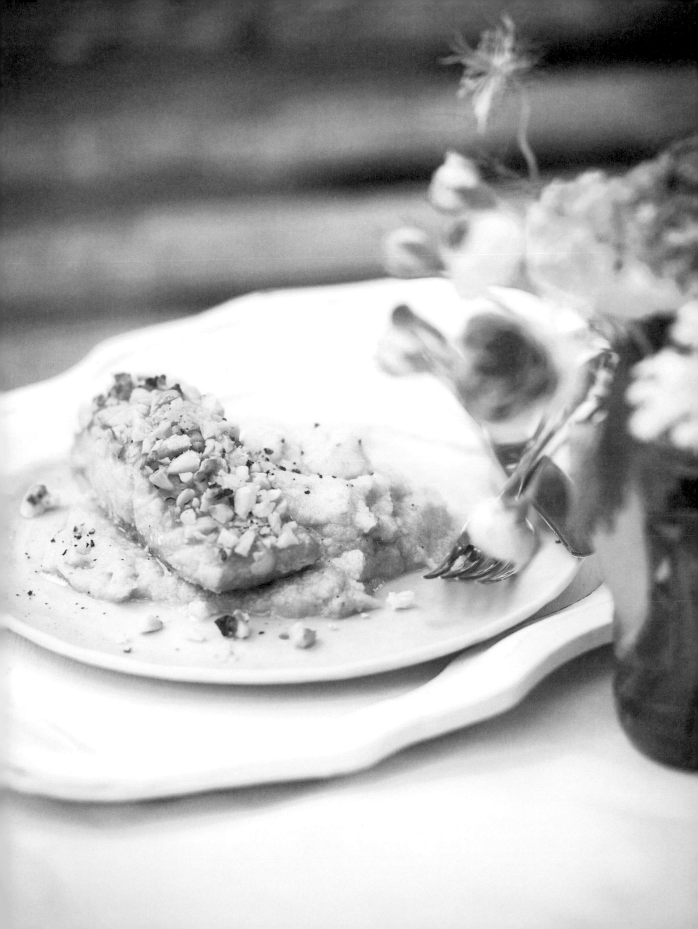

SPICED CHICKEN SAUTÉ WITH LEEKS & PEPPERS

Serves 2

4 boneless chicken thighs, skin removed and cut into bite-sized pieces (You can replace the thighs with 2 chicken breasts if you prefer. It will need less cooking time depending on the thickness of the breasts)

1 tbsp olive oil

1 red onion, finely sliced

2 leeks, finely sliced

2 peppers (red or yellow or mixture of both), diced

1 tbsp chickpea flour

300ml (½ pint) hot Chicken Broth (*see page 142*)

12 green olives (without flavour enhancers or preservatives), pitted

juice of ¼ lemon

sea salt and freshly ground black pepper

15 g chopped flatleaf parsley, to garnish

For the marinade

1 garlic clove, crushed

½ tsp smoked paprika

½ tsp ground turmeric

½ tsp ground cinnamon

½ tsp ground coriander

1 tsp ground cumin

1 tbsp olive oil

Mix all the marinade ingredients together in a large bowl. Add the chicken and toss to coat in the spice mixture. Cover with plastic film and let marinate in the fridge for a couple of hours or overnight.

Heat the oil in a large pan, add the onion and leeks and sauté over low for 15 minutes. Add the chicken and cook for 4–5 minutes, turning occasionally, until it is browned all over. Stir in the peppers, then sprinkle over the flour and add the broth and olives. Reduce the heat and simmer for 45 minutes. Stir in the lemon juice and then season with salt and pepper.

To serve, divide between serving plates and garnish with the parsley.

Vegetable dishes & salads

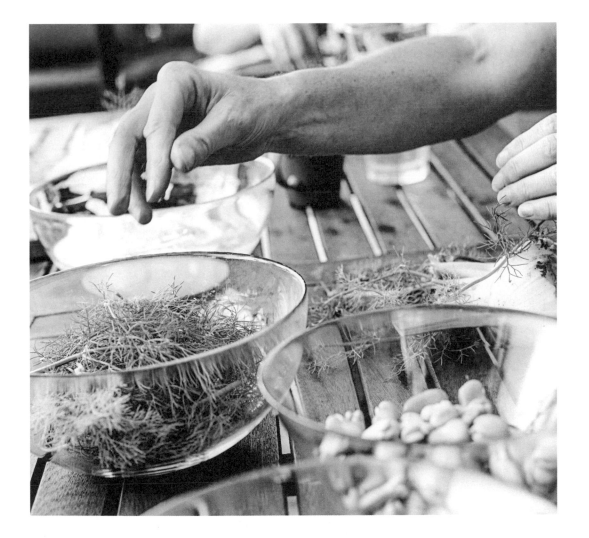

FRAGRANT AUBERGINES

Serves 2–3

4 tsp coconut oil

2 aubergines, cut into 5-cm
(2-inch) batons

5-cm (2-inch) piece fresh root
ginger, peeled and finely sliced

3 garlic cloves, finely sliced

1 small red chilli, finely sliced

4 spring onions, finely sliced

1 tbsp black glutinous rice wine,
such as Shaoxing rice wine

1 tsp brown rice vinegar

2 tsp dark soy sauce

2 tsp chickpea flour

1 tsp honey

100 ml (3½ fl oz) Chicken Broth
(*see page 142*) or vegetable broth

To garnish

1 handful fresh coriander leaves,
chopped

1 tbsp dried seaweed flakes

1 small red chilli, finely sliced

2 tsp black sesame seeds

Heat 3 teaspoons of oil in a wok or heavy-based pan, add
the aubergines, in batches if necessary, and cook over
medium–high heat for about 10 minutes until golden.
Remove from the pan and drain on kitchen paper.

Heat the remaining oil in the wok or pan, add the ginger
and cook over low heat until it changes colour but does not
char. Add the garlic, chilli and spring onions and cook for
a couple of minutes. Add the black and brown rice wines
and soy sauce. Whisk in the chickpea flour and honey and
then add the broth. Cook over high heat until the broth has
reduced by half. Reduce the heat, return the aubergines to
the wok or pan and cook gently until warmed through.

To serve, divide the aubergine mixture between plates
and garnish with the coriander, seaweed flakes, chilli and
sesame seeds.

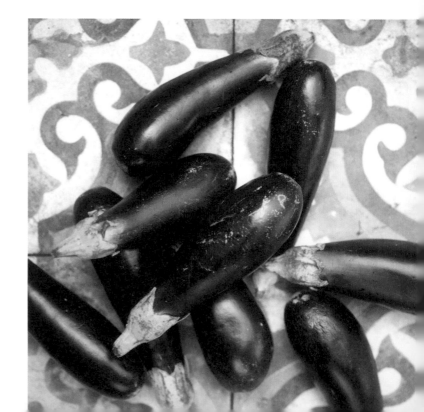

CAPONATA WITH TOASTED ALMONDS

Serves 2–3

1 aubergine, cut into 2-cm
(¾-inch) cubes

2 tbsp olive oil

1 red onion, chopped

2 celery sticks, finely chopped

1 garlic clove, crushed

1 x 400-g (13-oz) can chopped
tomatoes

1 tbsp red wine vinegar

2 tbsp capers

15–20 green olives (without flavour
enhancers or preservatives),
pitted

sea salt and freshly ground black
pepper

To garnish

1 heaped tbsp flaked almonds,
toasted

2 tbsp shredded mint

**You can make this a more substantial meal by serving
the caponata with a wholegrain of your choice and a
dollop of yoghurt.**

Preheat the grill to high.

Put the aubergine into a bowl with 1 tablespoon of oil and
toss to coat. Arrange the aubergines on a baking sheet
and grill for 4 minutes on each side, or until golden brown.
Set aside.

Heat the remaining oil in a large, heavy-based pan. Add
the onion and celery and sauté over a low heat for
10–15 minutes until soft and translucent. Add the garlic
and cook for 1 minute, then add the tomatoes and vinegar
and simmer for 40 minutes to allow the sauce to reduce a
little. Stir in the capers, olives and grilled aubergine, season
with salt and pepper, cover with a lid and simmer for an
additional 30 minutes.

Divide the caponata between serving plates and garnish
with the almonds and mint.

BUCKWHEAT SALAD WITH BUTTERNUT SQUASH, ASPARAGUS & PECANS

Serves 2

½ small butternut squash, peeled, seeded and cut into 1.5-cm (¾-inch) chunks

2 tbsp olive oil (or you could use 1 tbsp oil for roasting the butternut squash and 1 tbsp hemp oil for the dressing)

6 asparagus spears

50 g (2 oz) pecan nuts

100 g (3½ oz) buckwheat (or you could use freekeh instead)

1 small garlic clove, crushed

juice of ½ lemon

sea salt and freshly ground black pepper

Preheat the oven to 180°C/ 350°F/Gas Mark 4.

Place the butternut squash in a large roasting tin, drizzle over 1 tablespoon of oil and toss to coat. Season with salt and pepper. Roast in the oven for about 35 minutes until soft. Add the asparagus and pecans and roast for 8 minutes more. Let cool slightly.

Meanwhile, cook the buckwheat in a large pan of boiling water according to the packet instructions until tender. Drain well.

Transfer the buckwheat to the roasting tin with the vegetables, add the remaining oil and the garlic and lemon juice and toss gently. Serve hot or at room temperature.

Pecans are underappreciated but are high in immune-boosting manganese and also higher in antioxidants than other nuts.

BEETROOT & CHICKPEA FRITTERS WITH SAFFRON & MINT YOGHURT

Serves 2

2 raw beetroot, peeled and grated

1 carrot, grated

2 spring onions, finely sliced

115 g (3¾ oz) chickpea flour

¼ tsp ground turmeric

1 large handful fresh coriander leaves, finely chopped

2 eggs, lightly beaten

½ teaspoon sea salt

a generous grinding of black pepper

2 tbsp coconut oil or olive oil, for frying

mustard leaves, to serve

For the saffron & mint yoghurt

¼ tsp saffron threads

100 g (3½ oz) natural Greek yoghurt

1 tbsp extra virgin olive oil

juice of ½ small lemon

1 small garlic clove, crushed

2 tbsp chopped fresh mint

sea salt and freshly ground black pepper

First make the saffron & mint yoghurt. Put the saffron in a bowl, cover with 2 teaspoons of boiling water and let infuse for 5 minutes. Add the yoghurt, extra virgin olive oil, lemon juice and garlic and whisk together. Season with salt and pepper and then stir through the mint.

Using your hands, squeeze the grated beetroot over the sink to remove any excess water – I recommend that you wear rubber gloves to do this in order to avoid staining your hands.

Transfer the beetroot to a bowl, add the carrot, spring onions, flour, turmeric, coriander, eggs and salt and pepper and mix well to make the fritter batter.

Heat a dry frying pan and then add a little coconut oil or olive oil to form a thin layer over the bottom of the pan. Place 3 tablespoonfuls of the fritter batter into the pan. Fry the fritters over high heat for 2 minutes on each side, or until golden, gently pressing the fritters with a spatula to flatten them into discs while they cook. Transfer the fritters to a plate and keep warm while you cook the remaining batter.

Serve the fritters on a bed of mustard leaves with the saffron & mint yoghurt.

THREE-BEAN TAGINE WITH ALMOND & LEMON COUSCOUS

Serves 2

1 tbsp olive oil

1 large red onion, finely chopped

2 celery sticks, finely sliced

½ tsp ground cumin

¼ tsp cayenne pepper

¼ tsp smoked paprika

1 garlic clove, crushed

1 x 400-g (13-oz) can mixed beans, drained

400 ml (14 fl oz) passata

For the almond & lemon couscous

150 g (5 oz) couscous

½ tbsp olive oil

30 g (1¼ oz) flaked almonds, lightly toasted

½ preserved lemon, flesh removed and rind finely diced

sea salt and freshly ground black pepper

To garnish

2 tbsp chopped fresh coriander

2 tbsp natural yoghurt

This tagine is also really tasty if you serve it with a fried egg on top.

Heat the oil in a large, heavy-based pan. Add the onion and celery and cook over low heat for 15 minutes until soft and translucent. Add the spices and garlic and cook for 2 minutes, then stir in the beans and passata. Bring to the boil, then reduce the heat and cook over low heat for 45 minutes–1 hour until the sauce has thickened.

Meanwhile, make the couscous about 15 minutes before the tagine is ready to serve. Put the couscous into a pan with 150 ml (¼ pint) boiling water and the oil and stir well. Cover with a lid and let stand for 10 minutes. Stir the couscous with a fork to fluff up the grains, then stir in the almonds and preserved lemon. Season with salt and pepper.

Divide the tagine between serving plates, garnish with the coriander and a dollop of yoghurt and serve with the couscous.

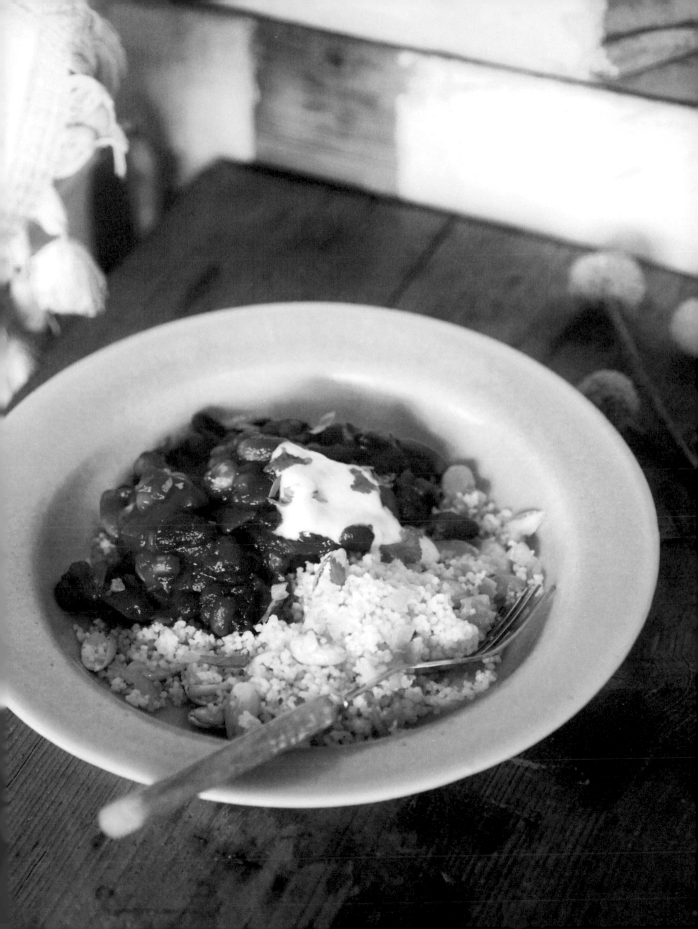

BEETROOT & COCONUT CURRY

Serves 2–3

1 tbsp coconut oil or ghee

1 large red onion, sliced

1 garlic clove, crushed

½ tsp ground turmeric

1 tsp black mustard seeds

1 tsp fenugreek seeds

300 g (10 oz) raw beetroot, peeled and cut into finger-sized batons

1 x 400-ml (14-fl oz) can coconut milk

2 tbsp natural Greek yoghurt

2 tbsp chopped fresh coriander, to garnish

Heat the coconut oil or ghee in a large, heavy-based pan. Add the onions and sauté over low heat for 15 minutes until soft and translucent. Add the garlic, turmeric and the black mustard and fenugreek seeds and cook for 2 minutes, then add the beetroot and coconut milk. Bring to the boil, then reduce the heat and simmer for 45 minutes, or until the beetroot is tender and the sauce has thickened. Stir through the yoghurt.

To serve, divide the curry between serving plates and garnish with the coriander.

GREEN BEAN STIR FRY WITH BLACK SESAME SEEDS

Serves 2–3

200 g (7 oz) green beans

1 tbsp olive oil

1 shallot, thinly sliced

2 garlic cloves, crushed

1 tbsp black mustard seeds

½ tsp chilli flakes

1 tsp grated unwaxed lemon zest

sea salt and freshly ground black pepper

First blanch the green beans. Fill a large bowl with iced water and set aside. Bring a large pan of water to the boil. Drop the beans into the boiling water and cook for 2 minutes. Drain, then plunge immediately into the iced water, then drain again thoroughly.

Heat the oil in a large, heavy-based pan. Add the shallot and garlic and sauté over high heat for 2 minutes. Add the mustard seeds, chilli, lemon zest and green beans and stir fry for 2 minutes until heated through. Season with salt and pepper and serve.

KIDNEY BEAN, QUINOA & LEEK SALAD WITH TOASTED PUMPKIN SEEDS

Serves 2

1 tbsp olive oil

2 leeks, finely sliced

125 g (4 oz) quinoa (use black quinoa if you can get it)

70 g (2¾ oz) rocket

80 g (3 oz) canned kidney beans, drained

1 handful pumpkin seeds, toasted, for sprinkling

For the dressing

5 tbsp hemp oil (or use extra virgin olive oil)

1 tbsp balsamic vinegar

1 garlic clove, crushed

½ preserved lemon, flesh removed and rind finely diced

sea salt and freshly ground black pepper

You won't need to use all the salad dressing for this recipe. Store any leftover dressing in an airtight container in the fridge and use within 5 days.

Heat the olive oil in a large frying pan, add the leeks and cook over low heat for 15 minutes, stirring constantly, until soft. Remove from the heat and let cool.

Cook the quinoa in a large pan of boiling water according to the packet instructions until tender. Drain well.

To make the dressing, whisk together the hemp oil, vinegar and garlic in a small bowl. Stir in the preserved lemon and season with salt and pepper.

To assemble the salad, put the leeks, rocket, kidney beans and quinoa into a salad bowl and gently mix together. Toss the salad with 2 tablespoons of the dressing and then sprinkle over the pumpkin seeds.

BUTTERNUT SQUASH, CHESTNUT & SEAWEED RISOTTO

Serves 2

½ small butternut squash, peeled, seeded and diced
3 tbsp olive oil
1 leek, finely sliced
1 red onion, finely sliced
500 ml (17 fl oz) Chicken Broth (*see page 142*) or vegetable broth
125 g (4 oz) risotto rice
10 roasted peeled chestnuts, finely sliced
2 tbsp flatleaf parsley, chopped
2 tsp dried seaweed flakes
sea salt and freshly ground black pepper
grated Parmesan cheese or vegetarian Parmesan-style cheese, to serve

Preheat the oven to 180°C/350°F/Gas Mark 4.

Place the butternut squash in a large roasting tin, drizzle over 1 tablespoon of oil and toss to coat. Roast in the oven for 30 minutes, or until soft.

Heat the remaining oil in a large, heavy-based pan. Add the leek and onion and cook over low heat for 15–20 minutes until soft and translucent.

Meanwhile, pour the broth into a pan and bring to the boil in a pan, them reduce the heat, cover with a lid and simmer gently while you make the risotto.

Add the rice to pan with the onion and leek and stir well. Add a ladleful of broth and cook over medium–high heat (you want the risotto to cook at a fairly high simmer), stirring frequently, until the broth has been absorbed by the rice, then gradually adding in more broth a ladleful at a time, making sure each addition is absorbed by the rice before adding the next ladleful. Repeat until there is only 1 ladleful of broth left and the rice is tender, about 25 minutes.

Add the roasted butternut squash, chestnuts, parsley, seaweed and the remaining broth, stir well to combine and cook until the broth has been absorbed. Season with salt and pepper, then remove from the heat and let stand for 5 minutes.

Divide the risotto between serving plates and serve with grated Parmesan or vegetarian Parmesan-style cheese.

WHITE BEANS WITH WILTED GREENS

Serves 2

200 g (7 oz) dried cannellini beans
a strip of kombu
1 bay leaf
piece of Parmesan cheese rind
 (optional – this will add a
 savoury note to the beans)
1 tbsp olive oil
1 large onion, finely sliced
2 celery sticks, finely chopped
1 garlic clove, thinly sliced
pinch of chilli flakes
3 anchovy fillets (optional)
100 ml (3½ fl oz) Chicken Broth
 (*see page 142*) or vegetable broth
300 g (10 oz) leafy greens, such as
 Swiss chard, spinach or dandelion
 leaves, shredded
100 g (3½ fl oz) rocket

To serve
fresh lemon juice
extra virgin olive oil
grated Parmesan cheese or
 vegetarian Parmesan-style cheese

Soaking the dried cannellini beans with a strip of kombu and then cooking them for a long time makes them much easier to digest. Anchovy fillets are a good source of omega-3 essential fatty acids but this dish will work just as well without them if you don't like the taste. If you are vegetarian you can replace the anchovies with 1 teaspoon dried seaweed flakes.

Soak the beans and kombu in a bowl of cold water for 6 hours or overnight. Rinse and drain the beans. Discard the kombu.

Put the beans into a large pan and cover with water. Add the bay leaf and the Parmesan rind, if using, and bring to the boil, then reduce the heat and simmer for 2–2½ hours until the beans are tender. Drain, discarding the bay leaf and Parmesan rind, if using, and set aside.

Heat the oil in a large, heavy-based pan, add the onion and celery and sauté over low heat for 15 minutes. Add the garlic, chilli and anchovies, if using, and cook for 2 minutes, stirring to break up the fish.

Lightly crush half the drained beans, then add the crushed and whole beans to the pan with the onion mixture. Pour over the broth and bring to a simmer, then add the leafy greens and rocket and simmer for 10 minutes.

Divide between serving plates, drizzle over a little lemon juice and extra virgin olive oil and serve with grated Parmesan or vegetarian Parmesan-style cheese.

BROCCOLI & QUINOA STIR FRY WITH AVOCADO & TOASTED ALMONDS

Serves 2

80 g (3 oz) quinoa

2 tbsp tamari soy sauce

1 tbsp toasted sesame oil

1 tsp brown rice vinegar

1 tbsp coconut oil

2 garlic cloves, crushed

2.5-cm (1-inch) piece fresh root
  ginger, peeled and grated

4 spring onions, sliced diagonally

300 g (10 oz) tenderstem broccoli

2 tbsp bean sprouts

1 tbsp black sesame seeds

To serve

cos lettuce leaves

1 avocado, peeled, stoned and
  thinly sliced

1 tbsp chopped fresh coriander

3 tbsp flaked almonds, toasted

Cook the quinoa in a large pan of boiling water according to the packet instructions until tender, then drain well.

In a small bowl, whisk together the soy sauce, sesame oil and vinegar and set aside.

Heat the coconut oil in a large frying pan or wok. Add the garlic, ginger, spring onions and broccoli and stir fry over high heat for 5 minutes. Add the bean sprouts and stir fry over high heat for 1 minute more. Add the quinoa and sesame seeds, pour over the dressing and mix well.

To serve, place a couple of lettuce leaves on each plate, spoon the stir fry into them and top with the avocado, coriander and almonds.

SPICED PANEER WITH WILTED GREENS

Serves 2

1 tbsp ghee or coconut oil

2 brown onions, finely chopped

2-cm (¾-inch) piece fresh root
    ginger, peeled and grated

2 garlic cloves, crushed

1 tsp ground turmeric

¼ tsp Kashmiri chilli powder

225 g (7½ oz) paneer, cubed

½ tsp sea salt

125 g (4 oz) Swiss chard, shredded

125 g (4 oz) spinach

4 tbsp natural yoghurt

100 ml (3½ fl oz) coconut water (or
    use filtered water)

1 handful fresh coriander leaves,
    chopped, to garnish

**This dish is good served with a grilled spiced chicken
breast or as a vegetarian meal with brown rice.**

Heat the ghee or coconut oil in a pan. Add the onions and
ginger and sauté over low heat for 15 minutes, then add
the garlic and cook for 2 minutes more. Stir in the turmeric,
chilli and paneer, making sure the paneer is well coated
with the spices, then add the salt, Swiss chard, spinach,
yoghurt and coconut water. Cover with a lid and cook over
high heat until the liquid is bubbling, then reduce the heat
and cook over low heat for 10 minutes.

To serve, divide the paneer between serving plates and
garnish with coriander.

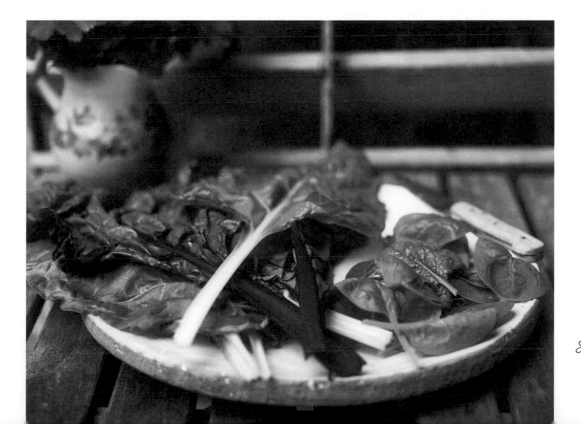

SWEET POTATO & CHICKPEA GNOCCHI

Serves 2

1 sweet potato, about 300 g (10 oz)
80 g (3 oz) chickpea flour, plus
   extra for dusting
40 g (1½ oz) ground almonds
1 egg yolk
¼ tsp ground nutmeg
sea salt
butter or Walnut & Rocket Pesto
   or Brazil Nut & Rocket Pesto (*see
   page 166*), to serve

FREEZING GNOCCHI

*These gnocchi freeze really
well, so they are ideal if you
like to cook large batches or
cook in advance. To freeze,
spread out the gnocchi in
a single layer on a baking
sheet and freeze for 2 hours,
then transfer portions of
gnocchi to freezer bags
and store in the freezer
for up to 1 month. To
reheat, cook as above but
increase the cooking time
to 4–5 minutes, allowing
the gnocchi to cook for
2 minutes after they have
risen to the surface.*

Preheat the oven to 200°C/400°C/Gas Mark 6.

Prick the skin of the sweet potato with a fork. Bake the
sweet potato in the oven for 45 minutes, or until soft.
Allow to cool slightly, then peel and discard the skin.

Put the sweet potato flesh into a bowl, season with a little
salt and mash with a fork. Using a wooden spoon, beat
in the flour, almonds, egg yolk and nutmeg. Transfer the
mixture to a freezer bag and chill in the fridge for 2 hours.

Divide the dough into 4 pieces. On a generously floured
work surface, roll each piece into a long sausage about
2.5 cm (1 inch) thick and then cut each roll into 2.5-cm
(1-inch) pieces. Lightly press the tines of a fork onto each
piece of gnocchi to create an indented striped pattern.

Bring a large pan of salted water to the boil. Cooking the
gnocchi in batches if necessary, drop the gnocchi into the
pan and cook for 2–3 minutes until they rise to the surface.
Remove the gnocchi with a slotted spoon and transfer to a
serving bowl.

Toss the gnocchi with some butter or pesto, divide between
serving plates and serve immediately.

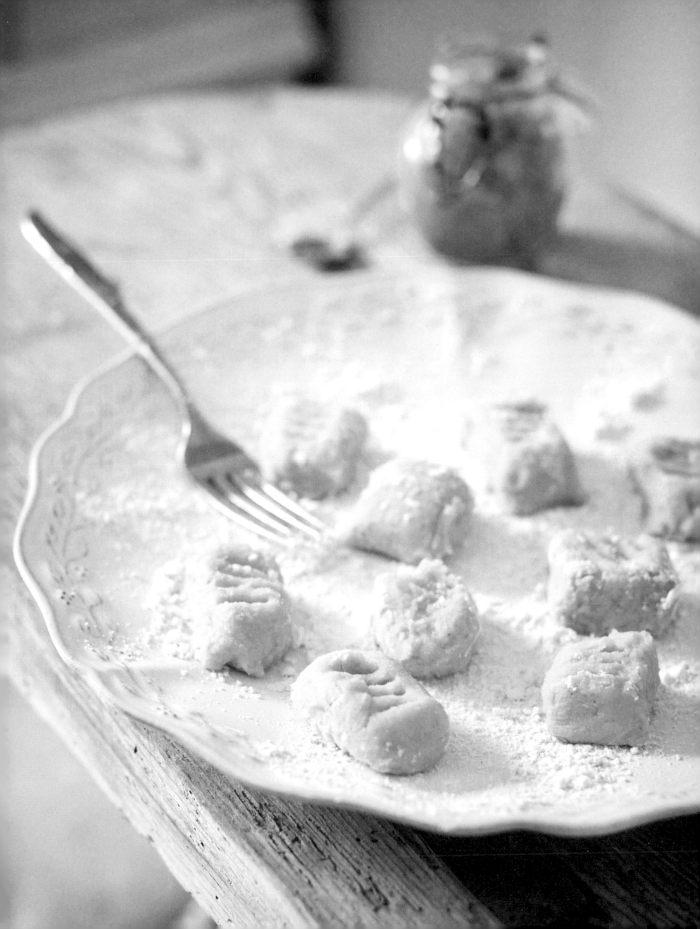

BAKED FETA WITH VEGETABLE SPAGHETTI

Serves 2

1 tbsp black sesame seeds
1 tbsp Nut, Spice & Seed Mix
  (*see page 168*)
1 x 200-g (7-oz) block feta cheese
1 tbsp honey

For the vegetable spaghetti
1 carrot, peeled
1 raw beetroot, peeled
1 courgette
1 tbsp olive oil
1 garlic clove, crushed

Change the vegetables you use to make the spaghetti according to the season – asparagus works well and provides prebiotic fibre. If you don't have the time or ingredients to make the nut, spice & seed mix, just double the quantity of black sesame seeds.

Preheat the oven to 200°C/400°C/Gas Mark 6.

Heat a dry frying pan until hot, then add the sesame seeds and toast for a couple of minutes until they are fragrant. Transfer to a shallow bowl and mix with the nut, spice & seed mix.

Using a pastry brush, coat the feta with the honey and then roll the feta in the sesame seed mixture. Wrap the feta in foil and place on a baking sheet. Bake in the oven for 10–12 minutes until the feta feels soft to the touch.

Meanwhile, using a spiraliser fitted with the thin noodle blade, spiralise the carrot, beetroot and courgette. Alternatively, use a vegetable peeler to cut the vegetables into ribbons.

Heat the oil in a wok or large frying pan. Add the spiralised vegetables and garlic and gently sauté over medium heat for 2–3 minutes until tender.

To serve, cut the feta into cubes, then divide the vegetable spaghetti between plates and sprinkle over the feta.

Sweet treats & drinks

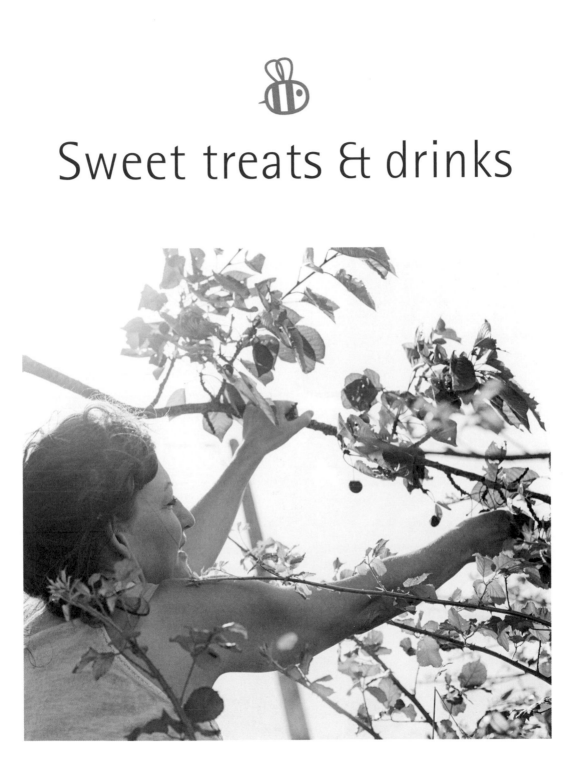

KEFIR PANNA COTTA WITH CARDAMOM & HONEY

Serves 8

3 gelatine leaves
120 g (4 oz) clotted cream
1 tbsp honey
1 vanilla pod, split in half
   lengthways and seeds scraped
   out
½ tsp ground cardamom
350 ml (12 fl oz) kefir

To serve
2 tbsp lemon curd
seasonal berries

Soak the gelatine leaves in a bowl of iced water for 5 minutes, or until soft, then squeeze it dry.

Meanwhile, put the clotted cream, honey and vanilla seeds into a small pan and cook over low heat for 5 minutes, whisking all the time. Remove from the heat, add the gelatine and cardamom and stir until the gelatine has melted.

Slowly pour in the kefir in a slow, steady stream, whisking continuously. Pour into 4 small glasses and leave to set in the fridge overnight.

Serve the panna cotta with seasonal berries and a little lemon curd.

VEGETARIAN OPTION

You can make a vegetarian version of this dessert by using agar-agar instead of gelatine. Put 1 tablespoon of agar-agar into a pan with 3 tablespoons of water and bring to the boil, then add the clotted cream, honey and vanilla seeds and simmer briskly for 5 minutes. Slowly pour in the kefir in a slow, steady stream, whisking continuously. Pour into 4 small glasses and leave to set in the fridge overnight.

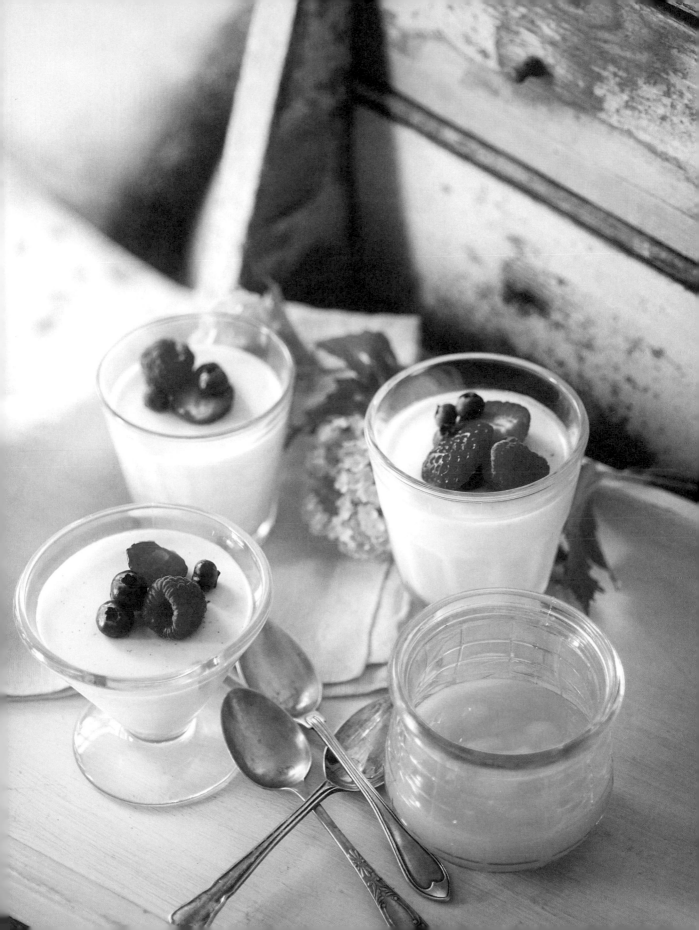

LEMON KEFIR CHEESECAKE

Serves 8

For the base

coconut oil, for greasing

100 g (3½ oz) walnuts

75 g (3 oz) brazil nuts

200 g (7 oz) Medjool dates, pitted

½ teaspoon pink Himalayan salt

For the filling

150 g (5 oz) Kefir Cheese (*see page 163*)

250 g (8 oz) ricotta cheese

100 g (3½ oz) honey

1 tbsp powdered gelatine

1 vanilla pod, split in half lengthways and seeds scraped out (or you could use ½ tsp vanilla extract)

juice and zest of 1 unwaxed lemon

1 tsp ground cardamom

300 ml (½ pint) thick double cream

To decorate

20 g (¾ oz) plain chocolate (70 per cent cocoa solids), grated

150 g (5 oz) raspberries

Lightly brush coconut oil over the base of a 22-cm (8½-inch) round loose-bottomed cake tin.

Put the walnuts, brazil nuts, dates and salt into a food processor and blitz until the mixture resembles fine crumbs. Spread the mixture evenly inside the prepared tin and press firmly to make the base for the cheesecake. Chill in the fridge or freezer while you prepare the filling.

Now make the filling. Put the kefir cheese, ricotta, honey, gelatine, vanilla seeds, lemon zest and juice and cardamom into a large bowl and whisk together for about 2 minutes until well blended. Gently fold the cream into the mixture. Spread the filling over the base and chill in the fridge for at least 2 hours.

When you are ready to serve, sprinkle the chocolate over the top of the cheesecake and decorate with the raspberries.

VEGETARIAN OPTION

To make a vegetarian version of the cheesecake filling, put the kefir cheese, ricotta, honey, gelatine, vanilla seeds, lemon zest and juice and cardamom into a large bowl and whisk together for about 2 minutes until well blended. Put 2 tablespoons of agar-agar into a pan with 50 ml (2 fl oz) water and bring to the boil, then simmer briskly for 5 minutes. Add the agar-agar to the bowl with the kefir cheese mixture and mix well, then gently fold the cream into the mixture.

SWEET CHESTNUT CONGEE

Serves 2

100 g (3½ oz) short, medium or
 long grain white rice (but not
 basmati rice)
8 roasted peeled chestnuts, sliced
2 tsp black sesame seeds
1 tsp white sesame seeds
½ tsp ground cinnamon
¼ tsp ground ginger

To serve

a little honey
2 tbsp flaked almonds, toasted, to
 sprinkle

Congee is a rice porridge that is made by slowly cooking rice in a large quantity of water until it breaks down and becomes a thick, creamy liquid. This cooking method softens and breaks down the rice so that it becomes easy to digest, making it very nourishing and healing. Try serving sweet congee with warmed stewed fruit for breakfast or make a savoury version (see box, below) for a nourishing evening meal.

Put the rice to a large, heavy-based pan with 500 ml (17 fl oz) filtered water and bring to the boil, then reduce the heat to low. Add the chestnuts and simmer for 30 minutes–1½ hours, stirring occasionally to prevent the rice sticking to the bottom of the pan, until the congee is your desired consistency. If you prefer your congee to have a soupy consistency, add a little more water if necessary. Remove from the heat and stir in the sesame seeds, cinnamon and ginger.

To serve, sweeten the congee with a little honey and sprinkle over the almonds.

SAVOURY CHESTNUT CONGEE

Follow the recipe above, replacing the honey and almonds with a little soy sauce, to taste, and 1 teaspoon of toasted sesame oil.

PROBIOTIC RASPBERRY, ROSE & CARDAMOM JELLIES

Serves 6

150 g (5 oz) raspberries
1 tsp rose water
1 tsp vanilla extract
½ tsp ground cardamom
2 tbsp gelatine powder
235 ml (7½ fl oz) kefir

Put the raspberries into a small pan and cook over low heat for 5 minutes, mashing the raspberries with a wooden spoon to make a sauce. Add the rose water, vanilla and cardamom and stir well. Remove from the heat.

Put the gelatine into a small bowl with 235 ml (7½ fl oz) warm water and mix well until the gelatine has dissolved.

Stir the gelatine mixture into the raspberry sauce and let stand for 5 minutes. Add the kefir and mix well. Pour into a small 22 x 10-cm (8½ x 4-inch) silicone mould and chill in the fridge for 1–2 hours until set.

Invert the jelly on to a chopping board and cut it into 6 slices. Alternatively, cut the jelly into 12 squares to be eaten as a snack. The jelly can be stored in an airtight container in the fridge for up to 4 days.

VEGETARIAN OPTION

Follow the recipe above to make the raspberry sauce with rose water, vanilla and cardamom. Put 2 tablespoons of agar-agar into a pan with 235 ml (7½ fl oz) water and bring to the boil, then simmer briskly for 5 minutes. Remove from the heat and let cool for 5 minutes. Stir the agar-agar into the raspberry sauce and let stand for 5 minutes, then continue as above.

DATE & BRAZIL NUT CANNONBALLS

Makes 10–14

140 g (4½ oz) dried pitted dates
  (see *tips on page 210*)
70 g (2¾ oz) brazil nuts
60 g (2½ oz) desiccated coconut
30 g (1¼ oz) raw cacao powder
2 tsp coconut oil
¼ tsp ground cinnamon
20 g (¾ oz) hemp seeds (or you
  could use desiccated coconut if
  you prefer)

Put the dates, brazil nuts, coconut, cacao, coconut oil and cinnamon into a food processor and blend until the mixture forms a thick paste.

Using your hands, roll portions of the mixture into bite-sized balls. Put the hemp seeds into shallow dish, then roll the cannonballs in the seeds to coat.

These snacks can be stored in an airtight container for up to 1 week.

ALMOND, APRICOT & COCONUT CANNONBALLS

Makes 10–14

140 g (4½ oz) dried pitted apricots
  (see *tips on page 210*)
60 g (2½ oz) desiccated coconut
60 g (2½ oz) ground almonds
2 tsp coconut oil
¼ tsp ground cinnamon
2 tsp white sesame seeds
2 tsp chia seeds (or omit this and
  double the quantity of sesame
  seeds)

Put the apricots, coconut, almonds, coconut oil and cinnamon into a food processor and blend until the mixture forms a thick paste.

Using your hands, roll portions of the mixture into bite-sized balls. Put the sesame and chia seeds into shallow dish, then roll the cannonballs in the seeds to coat.

These snacks can be stored in an airtight container for up to 1 week.

SPICED DATE & ALMOND CANNONBALLS

Makes 10–14

140 g (4½ oz) dried pitted dates
100 g (3½ oz) ground almonds
2 tsp coconut oil
½ tsp ground ginger
½ tsp ground cinnamon
¼ tsp ground green cardamom
20 g (¾ oz) white sesame seeds (or use a mixture of black and white sesame seeds)

Put the dates, almonds, coconut oil, ginger, cinnamon and cardamom into a food processor and blend until the mixture forms a thick paste.

Using your hands, roll portions of the mixture into bite-sized balls. Put the sesame seeds into shallow dish, then roll the cannonballs in the seeds to coat.

These snacks can be stored in an airtight container for up to 1 week.

TIPS

I use a Nutribullet to blend the ingredients but a regular food processor will work just as well.

Soaking the dried fruit in water, and adding a little of the soaking liquid to the ingredients, will make them easier to blend.

If you are tempted by chocolate, try adding a heaped teaspoon of raw cacao powder to the ingredients to help you combat your cravings.

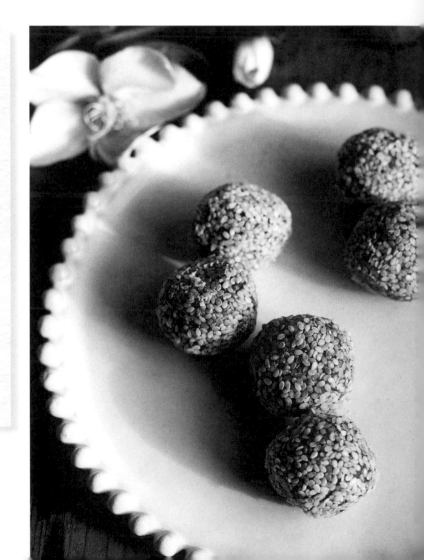

KEFIR YOGHURT POT

Serves 1

75 ml (3 fl oz) kefir
1–2 tsp chia seeds

To serve
a little honey
chopped nuts

This sweet yoghurt-like treat can be eaten as a snack or served for breakfast. The chia seeds are a good source of omega-3 essential fatty acids, protein and fibre.

Pour the kefir into a ramekin and stir in the chia seeds. Let soak in the fridge overnight – the chia seeds will swell up overnight to give the kefir a yoghurt-like consistency.

The next day, drizzle a little honey over the kefir, sprinkle with the nuts and serve.

AVOCADO KEFIR LASSI

Serves 2

1 tbsp chia seeds
400 ml (14 fl oz) kefir
1 ripe Hass avocado, peeled and
   stoned
½–1 tsp peeled and grated fresh
   root ginger (optional)
¼ tsp ground cumin
4–6 mint leaves

Kefir is a cultured milk product that provides probiotic organisms and a range of vitamins, minerals and amino acids. For people who are lactose intolerant it may improve lactose digestion and is a good way of increasing the amount of full-fat dairy in your diet. This drink provides healthy fats including omega-3 essential fatty acids from the chia seeds and the avocado, which is also a rich source of carotenoids. For a mango kefir lassi, substitute the avocado for a ripe mango.

If you have time, put the chia seeds into a bowl with the kefir and let soak at room temperature for 30 minutes – this will make the drink smoother.

Put all the ingredients into food processor or blender and process until smooth.

Pour the lassi into 2 glasses and serve immediately.

NOURISHING COCONUT, DATE & ALMOND DRINK

Serves 2

10 dates, pitted
300 ml (½ pint) coconut milk
½ tsp peeled and grated fresh root
    ginger
¼ tsp ground cinnamon
¼ tsp ground cardamom
a few drops of vanilla extract
1 tsp almond butter

If you are finding it difficult to give up caffeine you could try replacing your morning coffee with this rich, nourishing drink. Alternatively, the warming spices make it a soothing evening beverage.

Put all the ingredients into food processor or blender and process until smooth.

Pour the drink into 2 small glasses over ice and serve immediately or chill in the fridge until required.

TURMERIC MILK

Serves 2

500 ml (17 fl oz) milk (or substitute
    coconut milk or almond milk)
1 tsp grated turmeric root
1 cinnamon stick
4 cardamom pods
pinch of freshly ground black
    pepper
½ tsp peeled and grated fresh root
    ginger
a little honey

Put the milk, turmeric, cinnamon, cardamom, pepper and ginger into a small pan and cook over a medium heat, whisking all the time, until warmed through.

Pour the tea through a tea strainer into 2 glasses. Stir in a little honey to sweeten the drink and serve immediately.

BEET KVASS

**Makes 7 portions (enough for
1 person for a week)**

3 medium or 2 large raw beetroot
2 tsp sea salt
3 tbsp Whey (*see page 163*)

Beet kvass is a traditional Russian and Ukrainian fermented drink. Beetroot provides a good source of iron and folate and it is rich in phytonutrients. The nitrates in beetroot help the body to produce nitric oxide, which helps blood vessels dilate and improves blood flow. Beetroot also increases gut motility and is an excellent natural cure for constipation, making this probiotic drink an excellent blood and gut health tonic. If you prefer, you can omit the whey and double the quantity of salt.

Clean and trim the beetroot if they are organic; peel the beetroot if they are not organic. Cut the beetroot into 1-cm (½-inch) cubes.

Place the beetroot in a sterilised 750-ml (1¼-pint) jar (*see page 139*). Add the salt and whey and fill the jar with filtered water to within 2.5 cm (1 inch) of the top. Cover with a tight fitting lid and shake well. Let stand at room temperature for 2–3 days.

Strain the contents of the jar through a sieve into a bowl and discard the beetroot. Store the kvass in the fridge and drink as a daily tonic – it will keep in the fridge for 1 month.

To serve, pour a little kvass into a glass and top with filtered water.

Glossary

Chinese medicine

My love for this system of medicine has spanned 25 years; it has helped me help myself, my children, relatives, people who have bought my books and countless patients. I stand on the shoulders of giants when I attempt to pass some of it on to you. I hope that if you like what you see you will be inspired to read more on the subject. I would encourage you to seek out practitioners of Chinese medicine who use the tongue and the pulse and differential diagnosis to assess your conditions. It is no small task to simplify Chinese medicine and it is impossible to do it without some compromise. But, for the sake of conveying some basic ideas, I hope I will be forgiven for any oversimplification.

Blood: Blood circulates around the body much like the normal blood that is transported in our veins. When used with a capital B it refers to the Chinese medicine idea of Blood that has wider meaning and influence. Blood in the Chinese medicine sense is central to fertility and has a wide-reaching influence on menstruation, cycles, pregnancy and also the Heart and Spirit of a person. It is vital for fertility that Blood does not become deficient or depleted. Blood is made through good food, good digestion, adequate rest and by avoiding overwork, over-exercise and exhaustion. A weakness or deficiency in Blood may also come about after heavy blood loss or prolonged and heavy periods. Lack of Blood impacts on fertility in a number ways, including egg development, endometrial development and regular cycles.

Cold: Cold is a pathogenic factor that can predominate when we are exposed to cold environmentally or through an over-consumption of cold energy foods or through medication. For example, people who work in cold conditions, even supermarket workers who work where fridges and freezes emit cold air into the environment. Too much Coldness in the body slows down metabolism, may enable fluids to accumulate, creates heaviness, numbness, obstruction and low energy. In terms of fertility, too much Cold can prevent implantation and cause a general condition of obstruction and lack of flow. Traditionally a Cold womb was said to be inhospitable for an implanting embryo.

Damp: Dampness is a pathogenic factor that accumulates in the body either through exposure to Dampness in the environment or through consumption of Damp-forming foods. Infections, particularly STDs, cause Dampness to form in the body. Dampness frequently combines with either Heat or Cold to form Damp-Heat or Damp-Cold. In terms of fertility, it can impact on ovarian function, block tubes or create a hostile environment preventing implantation.

Dryness: An internal condition brought about through too little moisture; it is closely related to not enough Blood or not enough Yin. It can be due to becoming dehydrated, not consuming enough fluids or because the system is unable to take in fluids adequately. When there is Dryness predominating in the body, fertility is affected as the egg development may be affected, Heat may increase, the lining of the endometrium may also be compromised and cervical secretions dry out.

Essence: Another word for Jing.

Fire: An extreme form of Heat, where fluids are depleted. See *Heat* and *Dryness*.

Heat: A pathogenic factor that can come about through exposure to environmental heat, hot weather, toxins, chemicals, radiation, etc. Heat is generated through stress and working out in hot conditions. It is generated through the over-consumption of Hot foods, alcohol, drugs or medication. Warmth is very important for fertility but too much Heat can impact on the Blood and makes the Blood spill over and out of the vessels. In terms of fertility, this can impact on the way the Blood flows through the placenta and can impact on implantation. It may also mean that eggs develop too quickly and the cycles are short and the eggs immature preventing fertilisation.

Jing: The basis of life and reproduction. In many ways this book is about cultivating strong and abundant Jing in order to be more fertile! There are two types of Jing: the Jing we inherit from our parents and the Jing that we cultivate through the food we eat and the lifestyle choices that we make, as well as what happens to us in our life in terms of accidents and illness, etc. The stronger the Jing the stronger the reproductive capacity, and this will be manifested through our resilience to injury and illness, our energy, our vitality and our fertility.

Phlegm: An advanced state of too much Dampness. Often present in PCOS or blocked fallopian tubes.

Qi: Vital energy, life force, the impetus behind all life and movement. Qi runs through the meridians in our body influencing all bodily functions. A weakness, lack of or deficiency of Qi leads to illness and imbalance. The aim of an acupuncturist or a Qi gong master is to restore balance in the body through the movement and cultivation of Qi around and in the body. It is also one of the aims of this book. If you have strong Qi that flows well then your resistance to illness and injury will be better and your body will adapt better to challenging situations. Life is energy and energy is manifested in different forms in every living thing. Energy flows through our bodies in channels or meridians. Trees have energy, animals have energy, as do the Milky Way and the stars. Everything is Energy in various different expressions and intensity.

Stagnant Blood: a progression from Stagnant Qi or from injury. Sometimes when Cold predominates this can progress to a Stagnation of Blood. Pains in the body that are fixed or stabbing are due to Stagnation of Blood. Fibroids and endometriosis are all due to Stagnation of Blood. Retained products or scarring is also classified as Stagnation of Blood.

Stagnant Qi: This describes a situation where Qi does not flow well around the body and becomes stuck and stagnant. This may be experienced as pain or irregularity. Irregular periods or painful periods often point to a stagnation of Qi or symptoms that come and go. Emotionally being stuck and not getting where you want to in life may also cause Stagnation, manifesting as depression, inability to progress or envision your life clearly. Patients with this may also have digestive disturbance, bloating, gas, flatulence and they may also sigh a lot.

Yang: The motivating force in our body, it activates, stimulates and warms the body. Lack of Yang in the body will result in Cold and lack of motivation either physically or emotionally. Adrenal fatigue is a typical sign of Yang deficiency as is hypothyroidism. It is important for fertility to have good Yang energy, to warm, motivate and activate all the bodily functions and to keep the emotional motivation and

engagement alive. Sperm is the ultimate manifestation of Yang, active, fast, penetrating and explosive.

Yin: The cooling, nourishing, moistening, sustaining aspect of our body. Lack of Yin in the body will lead to dryness and an empty heat. In terms of our fertility, Yin deficiency will result in poor egg development and quality and poor sexual and reproductive capacity. Over work, over-exercise, excessive sweating all deplete the Yin of the body, leading to a situation where the body is lacking in nutrients, parched and inhospitable. The egg is the ultimate manifestation of Yin, yielding, passive, receiving and moist.

Western medicine

Adhesions: Scar tissues that attach to the surfaces of organs.

AMH: Blood test that measures the level of anti-Müllerian hormone (AMH), a hormone that is released by your ovaries. This can be used to estimate a woman's ovarian reserve (egg supply) to give an indication of how much longer she will be fertile.

Andrologist: Specialist in men's reproductive issues.

Anovulation: Absence of ovulation (menstruation may still occur).

Anti-nuclear antibodies: Antibodies that target 'normal' proteins within the nucleus of a cell.

Anti-phospholipid antibodies (APLAs): Proteins that may be present in the blood and may increase your risk of blood clots or pregnancy losses.

Anti-sperm antibodies: Antibodies that attack the sperm cells; these can be produced by both men and women.

Antral follicle count: Used to predict a woman's IVF success rate and her likely response to ovarian stimulation.

Asherman's syndrome: Scarring in the uterus, usually from a previous procedure, for example a sharp curettage following miscarriage or to remove the placenta after giving birth, Caesarean section or surgery to remove fibroids or polyps.

Aspirin: May be prescribed alongside IVF to improve chances of conceiving.

Assisted hatching: A microinjection procedure that chemically dissolves the embryo surface to facilitate implantation.

Azoospermia: Absence of sperm in the seminal fluid, which might be due to a blockage or an impairment of sperm production.

Basal body temperature: Your body temperature taken as soon as you awake. Recorded daily, this can help determine when and if ovulation is taking place during your cycle.

Beta-hCG test (BhCG): Blood test to detect pregnancy.

Biochemical pregnancy (also known as chemical pregnancy): Positive hCG level in the blood that doesn't continue to rise and so does not lead to pregnancy.

Blastocyst: Fertilised egg developed for five or six days (until this time described as an embryo).

Blighted ovum (egg): An egg that is fertilised but fails to implant/survive in the uterus.

Bromocriptine (Parlodel): Medication used to lower prolactin levels.

Cancelled cycle: Discontinuation of the IVF cycle due either to poor response, no egg recovery or failed fertilisation.

Cervical mucus: Secretions produced by the cervix that vary in quantity and consistency throughout the month.

Clexane: Drug used to stop blood clots forming.

Clomifene (Clomid): Drug used to stimulate production of follicle stimulating hormone (FSH) and luteinizing hormone (LH), often used to treat women who are not ovulating.

Cultures: Tests for infections in men and women.

Ectopic pregnancy: When the fertilised egg implants outside of the uterus, usually in the fallopian tube, ovary or abdominal cavity.

Egg donation: When eggs are removed from one woman to be used by another.

Egg freezing: When a woman's eggs are collected and frozen for future use.

Embryo freezing: When embryos are frozen during the IVF process, either for potential future use or to give time for the body to prepare for implantation; i.e. eggs fertilised with sperm = embryo

Endocrine disruptors: Man-made chemicals that can interfere with normal hormonal function.

Endometriosis: Presence of uterine lining in areas outside of the uterus, including the fallopian tubes, ovaries and bowel.

Endometrium: Mucus membrane lining the uterus.

ERPC: Evacuation of retained products of conception.

Fallopian tube: Transports the eggs from the ovary to the uterus. Where fertilisation usually takes place.

Fibroid: Non-cancerous tumour in the uterus.

Follicle: Fluid-filled sac on the ovary, from which the egg is released at ovulation or collected during an IVF cycle.

Follicle-stimulating hormone (FSH): Hormone produced in the anterior pituitary gland that stimulated the ovary to grow a follicle.

Follicular phase: Phase of the menstrual cycle during which follicles develop (after a period, pre-ovulation).

FSH test: Test used to assess ovarian reserve.

Genetic screening (IVF): Analysis of chromosomes for abnormalities in the IVF process.

Gonadotropin: Hormone that stimulates the testicles to produce sperm and the ovary to produce an egg.

Hysterosalpingogram (HSG): X-ray of the fallopian tubes and uterus, done seven, eight or nine days before ovulation.

Hysteroscopy: Used to investigate potential causes of very heavy or irregular menstrual bleeding, and in some cases to treat scarring (for example Asherman's syndrome, endometriosis).

In vitro fertilization (IVF): Procedure by which eggs are removed from the ovaries and fertilised with sperm in a laboratory. The fertilized egg (embryo) is later placed in the woman's womb.

Intra-cytoplasmic sperm injection (ICSI): Injection of a single sperm directly into an egg in order to fertilise it. The fertilised egg (embryo) is then transferred to the woman's womb.

Intralipid: Fat emulsion that has been shown to lower the activity of NK (natural killer) cells.

Intrauterine insemination (IUI): Procedure to separate fast-moving sperm from more sluggish or non-moving sperm, which are then placed into the woman's womb close to the time of ovulation.

Laparoscopy: Surgical procedure used to investigate and treat some gynaecological conditions.

Lupus: Auto-immune condition, probably genetic in origin and mainly affecting females.

Luteal phase: Phase in the menstrual cycle after ovulation and before the period starts.

Luteinising hormone (LH): Hormone produced by the anterior pituitary gland that causes the egg to be released by the ovary and stimulates progesterone production. In the male, LH stimulates testosterone production.

Male factor infertility, male subfertility: When a couple's fertility problems are attributed to male factors.

Metformin: Used in the treatment of PCOS to stimulate ovulation.

Molar pregnancy: An unsuccessful pregnancy in which the placenta and fetus do not form properly and a baby does not develop.

Motility: Percentage of moving sperm in a semen sample.

MTHFR: Genetic abnormality in clotting, indicated in some miscarriages. Treated with high doses of folic acid and aspirin to thin the blood.

Natural killer (NK) cells: Immune-system cells that normally help the body fight infections. There is now an idea that in some women these cells may attack the fetus as though it is an invader. It is a contentious area, but some doctors do advise using drugs to suppress the action of NK cells.

Oestrogen: Female hormones produced by the ovaries.

Oligospermia: Low sperm count.

Oocyte: Egg produced by the ovaries (also: ovum, gamete).

Orthorexia: Unhealthy obsession with eating healthy food.

Ovarian cysts: Small fluid-filled sacs that grow on the ovaries.

Ovarian drilling: A surgical treatment that can trigger ovulation in women with polycystic ovary syndrome (PCOS).

Ovarian hyperstimulation syndrome (OHSS): Possible side effect of IVF, when ovulation is medically stimulated, resulting in swollen, painful ovaries and sometimes bloating from fluid retention in the abdomen or chest.

Ovarian reserve: The age or health of the ovaries and eggs they contain.

Pelvic inflammatory disease (PID): Inflammation in the pelvis, often caused by sexually transmitted diseases or infection.

Polycystic ovary syndrome (PCOS): Hormone-related condition that causes small, underdeveloped follicles to grow on the ovaries. If left unmanaged, it can cause problems with fertility, as ovulation is less likely to occur.

Post-coital test: Test to ensure the sperm is getting through the cervix, also checking for hostile mucus, signs of infection or acidity, altered cervical mucus (too thick), and antibodies, which may attack the sperm.

Pre-implantation genetic diagnosis (PGD): The genetic investigation of hereditary disorders in an embryo before implantation into the uterus.

Premature ovarian failure: Cessation of ovulation, otherwise known as early menopause.

Progesterone: Hormone secreted by the corpus luteum of the ovary after ovulation.

Prolactin: Hormone produced by the pituitary gland, the level of which may affect ovulation.

Prostatitis: Infection or inflammation of the prostate gland. May cause poor sperm count.

Reproductive immunology: Field of medicine specialising in the relationship between the immune system and fertility and pregnancy.

Secondary infertility: The inability to conceive or carry a pregnancy to term after having previously had a successful pregnancy.

Semen analysis: Evaluation of the number and quality of sperm and how well they move (motility and morphology).

Sharp curettage: Surgical procedure in which the cervix is expanded using a dilator and the uterine lining scraped with a curette.

Sperm freezing: When semen is ejaculated or retrieved and frozen for IVF or future use.

Tamoxifen: Drug commonly used in cancer treatment, and also in fertility treatment when there are ovulation problems, as it inhibits the production of oestrogen.

Testosterone: Hormone produced in the male testicles

Thrombophilia: Excessive blood-clotting condition.

Varicocele: Enlargement of small veins under one or both testicles.

Vasectomy: Surgical procedure for male sterilisation.

Vitrification: Fast freezing process for eggs.

Xenoestrogens: Compounds found in things like insecticides and pesticides that mimic oestrogen in the body and so can disrupt hormonal balance.

References

Fertility fundamentals

1 Veleva, Z., et al., 'High and low BMI increase the risk of miscarriage after IVF/ICSI and FET.' *Human Reproduction* (2008) 23 (4): 878–884. Available at: http://humrep.oxfordjournals.org/content/23/4/878.short

2 Frisch, Rose E., *Female Fertility and the Body Fat Connection* (University of Chicago Press, 2003)

3 Maconochie, N., Doyle, P., Prior, S. and Simmons, R., 'Risk factors for first trimester miscarriage – results from a UK-population-based case-control study.' Department of Epidemiology and Population Health, London School of Hygiene & Tropical Medicine (2007)

4 Clark, A., et al., 'Weight loss in obese infertile women results in improvement in reproductive outcome for all forms of fertility treatment.' *Human Reproduction* (1998) 13: 1505

5 Rothschild, J., Hoddy, K., Jambazian, P., Varady, K., 'Time-restricted feeding and risk of metabolic disease: a review of human and animal studies.' *Nutrition Reviews* (2014) 308–318. Available at: http://dx.doi.org/10.1111/nure.12104

6 Gudmundsdottir, S., Flanders, W. and Augestad, L., 'Physical activity and fertility in women: the North-Trøndelag Health Study.' *Human Reproduction* (2009) 24 (12): 3196–204

7 Wise, L., Rothman K., Mikkelsen E., et al., 'A prospective cohort study of physical activity and time to pregnancy.' *Fertility & Sterility* (2012), 97 (5): 1136–42

8 Ignarro, L., Balestrieri, M. and Napoli, C., 'Nutrition, physical activity and cardiovascular disease: an update.' *Cardiovascular Research* (2007) 73: 326–40

9 Louis, G., Lum, K., Sundaram, R., et al. (2011). 'Stress reduces conception probabilities across the fertile window:

Evidence in support of relaxation', *Fertility & Sterility*, 95: 2184–89

10 Lynch, C., Sundaram, R., Maisog, J., et al., 'Preconception stress increases the risk of infertility: results from a couple-based prospective cohort study – the LIFE study.' *Human Reproduction* (2014), 29 (5): 1067–75

11 Campagne, D., 'Should fertilisation treatment start with reducing stress?' *Human Reproduction* (2006) 95: 2184–9

12 Eggert J., Theobald, H. and Engfeldt, P., 'Effects of alcohol consumption on female fertility during an 18-year period.' *Fertility & Sterility* (2004) 81: 379–83

13 Gill, J., 'The effects of moderate alcohol consumption on female hormone levels and reproductive function.' *Alcohol* (2000) 35 (5): 417–23

14 Juhl, M., Nyboe Andersen A. and Gronbaek, M., 'Moderate alcohol consumption and waiting time to pregnancy.' *Human Reproduction* (2001) 16 (12): 2705–9

15 Tolstrup, J., Kjaer, S., Holst, C., et al., 'Alcohol use as predictor for infertility in a representative population of Danish women.' *Acta Obstetricia Gynecologica Scandinavica* (2003) 82 (8): 744–9

16 Dechanet, C., Anahory, T. and Mathieu Daude, J., et al., 'Effects of cigarette smoking on reproduction.' *Human Reproduction* (2011) 17 (1): 76–95

17 American Society for Reproductive Medicine in collaboration with Society for Reproductive Endocrinology and Infertility, 'Optimising natural fertility.' *Fertility & Sterility* (2008) 90: 51–6

18 Bentzen, J., Forman, J., Larsen, E., et al., 'Maternal menopause as a predictor of anti-Müllerian hormone level and antral follicle count in daughters during reproductive age.' *Human Reproduction* (2012) 10: 1093

19 Waylen, A., Metwally, M., Jones, G., et al., 'Effects of cigarette smoking upon

clinical outcomes of assisted reproduction: a meta-analysis.' *Human Reproduction Update* (2009) 15 (1): 31–44

20 Anderson, K., Nisenblat, V. and Norman, R., 'Lifestyle factors in people seeking infertility treatment.' *The Australian & New Zealand Journal of Obstetrics & Gynaecology* (2010) 50: 8–20

21 Mueller, B., Daling, J., Weiss N., et al., 'Recreational drug use and the risk of primary infertility.' *Epidemiology* (1990) 1: 195– 200

22 Smith, C., 'Marijuana and the reproductive cycle.' *Science News* (1983) 123: 13

23 Battista, N., Rapino, C., Di Tommasoa, M., et al., 'Regulation of male fertility by the endocannabinoid system.' *Molecular & Cellular Endocrinology* (2008) 286S: S17–S23

24 Gold, M., Cocaine and Crack: *Neurobiology in Substance Abuse: A Comprehensive Textbook* 3rd edition (Williams & Wilkins: Baltimore, 1997)

Fertile food

1 Choy, C., Lam, C., and Cheung, L, 'Infertility, blood mercury concentrations and dietary seafood consumption.' *BJOG – An International Journal of Obstetrics and Gynaecology* (2002) 109 (10): 1121–5

2 Chalupka, S. and Chalupka, A., 'The impact of environmental and occupational exposures on reproductive health.' *Journal of Obstetric, Gynecologic, & Neonatal Nursing* (2010) 39 (1): 84–102

3 Nehra, D., Pan, A., Le, H., et al., 'Prolonging the female reproductive lifespan and improving egg quality with dietary omega-3 fatty acids.' (2012) *Aging Cell*, 11 (6): 1046–54.

4 Golding, J., Steer, C., Hibbein, J., et al., 'Dietary predictors of maternal prenatal blood mercury levels in the ALSPAC birth cohort study.' *Environmental Health Perspectives* (2013) 10: 1289

5 Wang, Q., Moly, K.H., 'Maternal diabetes and oocyte quality'. *Mitochondrion* (2010) 10 (5): 403–10

The menstrual cycle
1 Levitas, E., Lunenfeld, E. and Weiss, N., 'Relationship between the duration of sexual abstinence and semen quality; analysis of 9,489 semen samples'. *Fertility & Sterility* (2005) 83 (6): 1680–6.

Fertile in body-mind-gut
1 Hilimire, M.R., DeVylder, J. E., Forestell, C.A., 'Fermented foods, neuroticism, and social anxiety: An interaction model'. *Psychiatry Research* (2015) 228 (2): 203–8

2 Sharma, R., Biedenham, K., Fedor, J., et al., 'Lifestyle factors and reproductive health: taking control of your fertility'. *Reproductive Biology & Endocrinology* (2013) 11: 66.

3 Krishner, R., 'In vivo and in vitro environmental effects on mammalian oocyte quality'. *Annual Review of Animal Biosciences* (2012) 1: 393–417

4 Legro, R., Sauer, M. and Mottla G., 'Effects of air quality on assisted human reproduction'. *Human Reproduction* (2010) 25 (5): 1317–24

5 Selevan, S., Borkovec, L., Slott, V., et al., 'Semen quality and reproductive health of young Czech men exposed to seasonal air pollution'. *Environmental Health Perspectives* (2000) 108 (9), 887–894

6 Rubes, J., Selevan, S. et al., 'Episodic air pollution is associated with increased DNA fragmentation in human sperm without other changes in sperm quality'. *Human Reproduction* (2005) 20: 2776–83

7 Wolverton, B.C., Douglas, W.L., Bounds, K., 'A study of interior landscape plants for indoor air pollution abatement'. *NASA* (1989) NASA-TM-108061

Fertile eggs
1 Office of National Statistics (2012)

2 Royal College of Obstetricians and Gynaecologists (2009)

3 Center for Disease Control (2008)

4 Grasselli, F., Baratta, L., Baioni, I., Bussolati, S., et al., 'Bisphenol A disrupts granulosa cell function'. *Domestic Animal Endocrinology* (2010) 39 (1): 34–9

5 Ehrlich S., Williams, P.L, Missmer, S.A., Flaws, J.A., Berry, K.F.,Ye X., Calafat, A.M., Petrozza, J.C., Wright, D., Hauser, R, 'Urinary bisphenol A concentrations and early reproductive health outcomes among women undergoing IVF.' *Environmental Health Perspectives* (2012) 120 (7) 978–83

6 Fusi F.M., Ferrario, M., Bosisio, C., Arnoldi, M,. Zanga, I., 'DHEA supplementation in women with diminished ovarian reserve: a case control study'. *Reproductive Biology & Endocrinology* (2009) 7 (7): 108

7 Hyman J.H., Margalioth E.J., Rabinowitz R., Tsafrir A., Gal M., Alerhand S., Algur N., Eldar-Geva T., 'DHEA supplementation may improve IVF outcome in poor responders: a proposed mechanism'. *European Journal of Obstetrics, Gynecology & Reproductive Biology* (2013) 168 (1): 49–53.

8 Kara M., Aydin T., Aran T., Turktekin N., Ozdemir B., 'Does dehydroepiandrosterone supplementation really affect IVF-ICSI outcome in women with poor ovarian reserve?', *European Journal of Obstetrics, Gynecology & Reproductive Biology* (2014) 173: 63–5.

9 Fouany M.R., Sharara F.I., 'Is there a role for DHEA supplementation in women with diminished ovarian reserve?', *Journal of Assisted Reproduction & Genetics* (2013) 30 (9): 1239–44.

Fertile man
1 Chavarro, J.E., Toth, T.L., Sadio, S.M., Hauser, R., 'Soy food and isoflavone intake in relation to semen quality parameters among men from an infertility clinic'.

Human Reproduction (2008) [Epub ahead of print]

2 Jensen, T.K., Gottschau, M., Madsen, J.O.B., et al., 'Habitual alcohol consumption associated with reduced semen quality and changes in reproductive hormones; a cross-sectional study among 1221 young Danish men'. *The BMJ Open* (2014), 4 (9)

3 Paul, C., Murray, A., Spears, N., et al., 'A single, mild, transient scrotal heat stress causes DNA damage, subfertility and impairs formation of blastocysts in mice'. *Reproduction* (2008) 136:73–84.

4 Tiemessen C., Evers, J. and Bots, R., 'Tight-fitting underwear and sperm quality'. *The Lancet* (1996) 347: 1844 5

5 Kilgallon, S. and Simmons, L., 'Image content influences men's semen quality'. *Biology Letters* (2005) 1: 253–255

6 Avendaño, C., Mata, A., et al., 'Use of laptop computers connected to internet through wi-fi decreases human sperm motility and increases sperm DNA fragmentation'. *Fertility & Sterility* (2012) 97 (1): 39–45

7 Robbines, W., Xun, L., FitzGerald, L., et al., 'Walnuts improve semen quality in men consuming a western-style diet: randomized control dietary intervention trial'. *Biology of Reproduction* (2012). Available at: http://www.biolreprod. org/content/early/2012/08/07/ biolreprod.112.101634

8 Durairajanayagam, D., Agarwal, A., Ong, C., et al, 'Lycopene and male infertility'. *Asian Journal Andrology* (2014) 16 (3): 420–5

IVF support
1 Hoon, M.W., Johnson, N.A., Chapman, P.G., Burke, L.M., 'The effect of nitrate supplementation on exercise performance in healthy individuals: a systematic review and meta-analysis'. *International Journal of Sport Nutrition & Exercise Metabolism* (2013) 23 (5): 522–32

Index

Author acknowledgements
To women everywhere, nourishment starts with self.

To my family; Roger, Lily, Violet, my four sisters and my mother, Fay. Thank you for supporting me and for the thrill of taking the adventure of life together. Love is at the centre of all that drives me; love of life and love of family and friends. I would be nothing without your love.

To my amazing friend and co-writer Victoria Wells, without whom this book would not have been possible. Thank you for your friendship above all else.

To everyone at Ebury; Katy Denny, Anna Davidson McCrae, Clare Churly, Tracy Killick, William Shaw, Denise Smart, Jo Thorne, Juliet Percival, Tony Hutchinson, Sarah Bennie and Lucy Harrison.

To my team; Cathryn Summerhayes, Laura Hersch, Alison Smith, Michelle Hogg, Michelle Mazewski, and Kate Adams. You are the glue and the support that makes it all possible.

To all those people who have believed in me in my life; you have helped me believe in myself. And to those who have inspired and encouraged me; I thank you from the bottom of my heart. I stand on the shoulders of giants: my ideas and inspirations are channelled from researchers, physicians, healers, cooks and ordinary people. I am inspired by people who manifest and action their ideas, dreams, hopes and creativity, and bring them to the world, determined to make a difference. I am proud to carry on this tradition.

To all you amazing women who have trusted me with your most deeply held desire. I never take that trust for granted and I truly honour being the keeper of your stories. Go into the world and teach each other to be better at receiving, to value being fertile and to nurture children who understand that all love starts with self.

To my father, long gone, who taught me that we all have a unique gift and it is our duty to find it and bring it to the world.

Resources
If you are struggling to get pregnant, are planning on starting fertility treatment, or have questions about preserving your fertility then you can find out more about Emma Cannon's FERTILE support programme by visiting **www.emmacannon.co.uk.**

Team credits
Commissioning Editor **Katy Denny**

Managing Editor **Clare Churly**

Art Director **Tracy Killick** at Tracy Killick Art Direction and Design

Production Manager **Lucy Harrison**

Photographer **William Shaw**

Food Stylist **Denise Smart**

Prop Stylist **Tony Hutchinson**

Illustrator **Juliet Percival**

Publisher's acknowledgements

The publisher would like to thank Emma Cannon for kindly allowing us the use of her lovely home for the photoshoot; and the team at Mad Lilies in Banstead, Surrey, for supplying the beautiful flowers for the photoshoot. www.madlilies.co.uk.

Picture credits
Special photography by William Shaw.

Other photography:
Roger Cannon 4, 9. **Dreamstime** 2 Alexionas; 10 Mk 74; 24 Huhulin; 43 Lermun; 72 Freila; 109 Looby. **Shutterstock** 27 Casanisa 37 Chamille White; 53 Bykofoto; 82, 83, 84 Enraged; 85 Yunava1; 87 Vichailao; 88 Images72; 93 Zuender; 95 Zaira Zarotti; 96 Natasha Breen; 101 Sarah2; 105 gpoint-studio; 108 Ev Thomas; 118 Gayvoronskaya_Yana; 129 Lolostock. **Jo Thorne** 6, 10, 31, 33, 35, 36, 40, 49, 59, 63, 69, 121, 123 (all), 124, 141, 187, 203, 210.

Watercolour backgrounds, small illustrations and paper textures used throughout: **Shutterstock** Anno, Undrey, Maxim Ibragimor, Pun Photo, Nadezha Shlemina. **Dreamstime** Martina Vaculikova, Olena Tieriekhova, Aggressor, Flas 100.

Illustrations:
Bee illustrations used throughout courtesy **Emma Cannon**.

Juliet Percival 47, 67, 112.

Caerleon.
25/3/17.